Contents

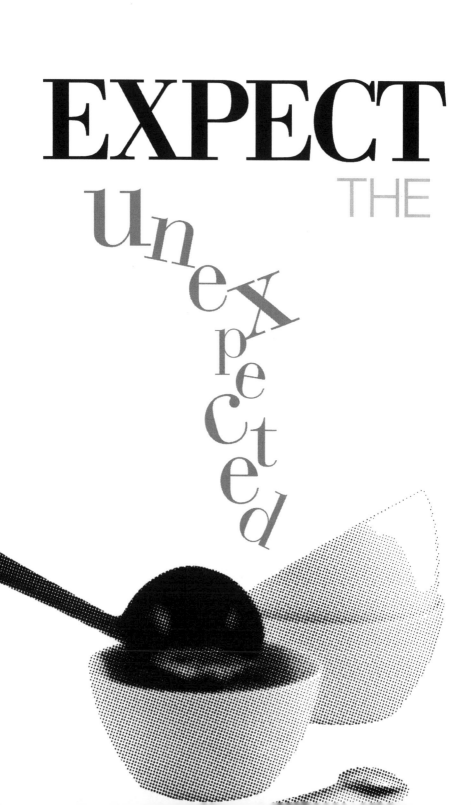

Have you ever come across a diet book that presents you with **'the diet'** in the first few pages? Probably not! But it makes a lot of sense. Dieters generally head straight to the diet plan with barely a glance at the introductory chapters so we are going to cut to the chase and give you our **10 Day Flab-Fighting Soup Diet** right here, which you can start immediately and see some serious fat loss before you even turn to the pages explaining **why** soup works for fast and lasting fat loss!

Of course, we hope you **will** read the whole book because it took months to research and write and more hours than we care to admit to devise, test and tweak the recipes. We also desperately want you to become a dedicated *soupaholic* (more about that later) but for now here are the main reasons why soup is superb for fat loss plus the diet programme.

It's a Miracle in a Bowl!

- Soup cuts calories.
- Soup fills you up.
- Soup blunts your appetite.
- Soup crushes cravings.
- Soup banishes bloating.
- Soup feeds stress.
- Soup balances hormones.
- Soup boosts metabolism.
- Soup keeps you sharp.
- Soup helps you sleep.

THE 10 DAY

FLAB-FIGHTING

SOUP DIET

First Thing in the Morning

Get up, get out and get physical before anyone else is up and you get sucked into the 'morning routine'. Exercising first thing in the morning burns more calories for up to eight hours and exercising for 30 minutes on an empty stomach is the way to go. Running, jogging or brisk walking not only gets the heart pumping but also delivers oxygen around the body which energises cells, pumps up the level of feel good endorphins and sets you up for a demanding day ahead. If it is cold, wet, windy, icy or downright depressing weather-wise, go to the gym or run up and down the stairs, skip or jog on the spot indoors, get the mini trampoline out and watch early morning TV while you bounce - just get your heart pumping for 30 minutes!

After Your Shower

Have a bowl/mug of one of the following soups (see recipe section):

- Gazpacho-Style Soup
- Very Quick Tomato Soup
- Light Chicken Soup
- Chinese Little Gem & Chicken/Tofu Soup

Soup for breakfast may be a totally alien concept to you but many Japanese and Koreans wouldn't leave home without it and they have amongst the lowest rates of obesity in the world. Protein and fat-rich soups play a major role in Scandinavian diets early in the day and they are also amongst the leanest people on the planet. So, don't get hung up on habit, give it a go and leave the house well-nourished and ready for what the morning might throw at you. If you are in a frantic rush, flask it. Buy yourself one of those large cup flasks that are usually meant for coffee and sup happily on your way to work, when you get there or if you are home-based, as soon as you get a moment to yourself.

If you really can't face soup this early in the day, go for one of the mid morning/mid afternoon snacks suggested below.

Mid Morning and/or Mid Afternoon

Have a bowl/mug of one of the following soups (see recipe section):

- Thai Curry Sweet Potato Soup
- Spinach & Watercress Soup
- Beef Broth with Pearl Barley

OR one of the following snacks:

- 2 oatcakes with tinned, mashed salmon topped with cucumber slices.
- A tray or pack of raw baby vegetables with a small pot of hummus, tzatziki or natural cottage cheese.
- A 3 Bean Salad from the deli (or make your own).
- A small pack of fresh nuts or a nut and seed mix and a piece of fresh fruit.
- 2 brown Ryvita or rye crackers with chopped boiled egg mixed with natural yoghurt and chopped fresh herbs.
- A couple of celery sticks filled with nut butter (almond, cashew, hazelnut, walnut, macadamia or peanut).
- A cold cooked chicken leg, breast or thigh (skin off) with a couple of tomatoes and a handful of fresh walnuts.
- A small pot of 0% fat Greek yoghurt topped with a handful of fresh berries and a good scattering of toasted, flaked almonds.
- Half an avocado filled with tinned tuna and a dollop of salsa.

Lunchtime

This is the time of day where soup is a **must** for fast fat loss. For now, don't question it, just do it and when you get a minute, read **why** later in the book. You may also need/want to add a salad to ensure you don't experience an energy dip an hour or so later.

Have a bowl/mug of one of the following soups (see recipe section):

- Thai Curry Sweet Potato Soup
- Spinach & Watercress Soup
- Beef Broth with Pearl Barley

Add a small mixed salad if needed. Lots of green leaves, lots of colour and dress with a good splash of olive oil and a little lemon juice. If you opt for a bought salad, go easy with the little pack of dressing. They often have rather a lot of sugar added and there is always more than you need.

Early Evening

For women in particular, this is a very dangerous time of the day. Our 'girlie' hormones way too often control our eating behaviour and they can have an exasperatingly-strong influence on how our hunger, appetite, blood sugar and stress hormones behave and the early evening 'munchies' can all-too-quickly be our undoing. Soup, however can be our saviour and just a cupful can make a huge difference and still the hormonal havoc!

Have a bowl/mug of one of the following soups (see recipe section):

- Gazpacho-Style Soup
- Very Quick Tomato Soup
- Light Chicken Soup
- Chinese Little Gem & Chicken/Tofu Soup
- Miso Soup (see Instant and Ready-Made Soups in the recipe section)

Evening Meal

It really depends on what you have had during the day whether you go for soup in the evening or opt for a decent portion of lean protein and a load of vegetables or a salad with a few important fats thrown in to satisfy your appetite. Here are your choices during the ten days:

Choose one of the following soups (see recipe section):

- Pea Mint & Lettuce Soup
- Spicy Meatball Soup

- Gazpacho-Style Soup
- Chinese Little Gem & Chicken/Tofu Soup

And/or select one of the following:

All suggestions make one serving. Pile your plate with a selection of steamed, roasted or stir fried vegetables (3 is a good number to aim for) or a good-sized mixed salad.

Very Quick Chicken

Steam a skinless chicken breast either on a plate (cover it loosely with tinfoil/greaseproof paper) over a pot of simmering water or in a steam basket for 10-15 minutes until cooked through. Spread pesto or olive paste on top and put under the grill (low heat) for a couple of minutes to warm through.

Very Quick Salmon

Lightly paint a salmon fillet or salmon steak with olive oil and grill under a moderate heat for 7-8 minutes, turning once. Sprinkle with Worcestershire Sauce or balsamic vinegar and lime or lemon juice just before serving.

Very Quick Fish

Grill or microwave a couple of white fish fillets until the fish flakes easily (4-6 minutes dependent on type and thickness of fish). Warm through a couple of tablespoons of tomato salsa while the fish is cooking. Top the fish with the salsa and sprinkle with chopped herbs, ground black pepper and lemon juice at the last minute.

Very Quick Lamb

Rub a lamb steak with lemon zest, a pinch of cinnamon and a splash of olive oil mixed. Grill under a moderate heat for 4 minutes each side if you like it pink, longer for well done. Put on a warm plate and leave to rest for a few minutes while you heat through a little fresh orange juice with very finely diced fresh red chilli (deseeded) then pour this over the lamb.

Very Quick Pork

Mix a spoonful of peanut butter with a little sweet chilli sauce and season with pepper. Put 2 thinly sliced pork fillets on a baking tray, brush the tops with half the nutty mixture and grill under a moderate heat for 2 minutes. Carefully turn the pork over, brush the other side with the remaining mixture then grill for another 2 minutes or until cooked through. Serve with fresh apple slices and chopped fresh coriander and/or mint.

Very Quick Mackerel
Bake a couple of smoked mackerel fillets (skin side down) in a medium hot oven until deliciously hot and smokey. About 4-5 minutes.

Very Quick Prawns
Coat half a dozen fresh, raw prawns with chilli, garlic or lemon-infused olive oil and grill both sides until pink but not dried out (2-6 minutes depending on the size of the prawns).

Very Quick Omelette
Preheat the oven to 190C/375F/Gas Mark 5 and lightly grease a small baking dish with olive oil. Beat 2 eggs in a bowl and add stuff from the fridge (see below for suggestions). Season with sea salt and freshly ground black pepper and pour into the prepared dish. Bake for 15-20 minutes or until the top is slightly golden and a knife inserted in the middle comes out clean. Let it cool for a few minutes before serving.

- Diced cold ham
- Sliced cold cooked chicken
- Grated Swiss cheese
- Finely chopped sweet peppers/artichokes/sun dried tomatoes in jars
- Freshly chopped parsley, basil or other herbs

Very Quick Tofu
Cut firm tofu into cubes and stir fry quickly in a little olive oil mixed with crushed garlic and grated fresh ginger. Add a squeeze of runny honey and top with toasted flaked almonds.

Very Quick Burger
Use freshly ground lean beef, lamb or soya mince (which has been soaked as per packet instructions). Add some sea salt crystals, ground

black pepper and other spices of choice (cumin, coriander, curry powder, chilli powder etc), plus a few shakes of Worcestershire Sauce or balsamic vinegar. Mould into burger shapes and chill for 15 minutes before grilling. Top with a slice of goats cheese cheddar towards the end of cooking until melted and bubbling.

Before Bed

Do not go to bed hungry or you are more than likely looking at blood sugar lows through the night, less than regenerating sleep and early to mid morning cravings for starches, sugars and stimulants the next day. If you are not hungry and sleeping well, there is no need. There is just one soup choice here but boy does it tick all the boxes, principally because it is rich in nutrients that encourage the production of the *calming* chemical, serotonin. You will discover as you read through the book that we discourage starchy carbohydrates after 6pm but the bedtime soup plays to different rules and there are good reasons why, which will be explained.

* Turkey/Tofu & Spinach Soup (see recipe section)

Drinks

When you are supping soup regularly during the day, both the water content and the vegetables will keep you pretty well-hydrated but there are plenty of other liquids you can include.

* Water of course, both still and sparkling.
* Fresh fruit juices mixed 50:50 with still or sparkling water.
* Fresh vegetable juices.
* Black, green and red bush tea (no milk or sugar).
* Good black coffee made with fresh beans (no milk or sugar).
* The occasional glass of dry white or good red wine or dry champagne if funds allow!
* Stay away from fizzy soft drinks - sugar, sugar, sugar and the *diet* and *zero* versions are no better - a quick look at the list of ingredients says it all!

Preparation and Cooking Tips

There are ten **SuperSkinny** soups and we urge you to include a good selection during the 10 days. Successful fat loss results when a variety of tastes, textures and foods are consumed; diet boredom should **not** be on the cards here. However, you may have favourites which is fine but aim for a minimum of four to five. Try to make time to prepare the soups in bulk and refrigerate and/or freeze in small portions to ensure you can 'grab and go'. There are also a few suggestions for **Instant and Ready-Made** soups in the **SuperSkinny Soups** part of the recipe section to get you out of trouble on those days where the plan threatens to go pear-shaped or you haven't had time to make soup.

More of the Unexpected!

We take a fairly global approach to our soups and invite you to be a bit adventurous and adopt an experimental approach. We believe you will quickly discover that you don't need, want or crave the Western 'staples' like cereals/toast for breakfast, sandwiches for lunch, pasta/potatoes/rice at dinner and sugary snacks and drinks that may currently invade your day.

Yes, there is a bit of slicing, dicing and cooking time involved but if you stock up on a few store cupboard essentials, have a small freezer, a blender, a slow cooker (a good investment when time is tight), a thermos flask and can manage a quick sweep around the supermarket once a week, our soups won't be time-consuming and labour-intensive. And more importantly, your day will not be invaded by hunger and cravings.

Important

This diet/way of eating is all about the fat busting properties of soup so after you have followed the **Flab-Fighting Soup Diet** for 10 days, soup should continue to feature in your life at least once a day. This is in no way a life devoted to liquids where a knife and fork never take the stage and when you get around to reading **why** soup can make you thin you will realise that it is *nutritional perfection in a bowl* because of the way the liquid works with the solids within the soup to aid digestion, nourish you and burn fat. Soup is fascinating stuff and we are keeping an eagle eye on proven and ongoing studies in an endeavour to keep you right up to date with its fat burning fabulousness.

So, let's get started. The soups can all of be made in bulk, portioned and kept in the fridge for a couple of days or frozen. If you find a bit of kitchen time therapeutic at the end of a busy day, make your soup and eat it while it is super-fresh and bursting with goodness but if you are more of a 'scant time to get into the kitchen' type, plan ahead and devote a morning/afternoon to making all the soup you need for your 10 days, bag and freeze them. As mentioned, you don't have to make them all - some dieters tell us they just stick to four or five over the 10 days and boredom doesn't set in but only you know how well (or badly) you cope with routine eating!

You don't have to follow the exact programme every day; repetition is great for exercise and learning French verbs but doesn't work so well for fat loss. Hunger won't be an issue so if you don't feel like eating first thing in the morning, don't force food down, similarly if you know you invariably suffer from energy dips mid afternoon get the flask out and dive in. The only *rule* is that you don't have the soups that contain starchy carbohydrates for your evening meal as you don't need the extra energy they provide at this time of the day unless you exercise in the evening, in which case the soups without starch may not fill you up. All the soup recipes clearly state whether starches are included or not.

WHY WE LOVE
SOUP

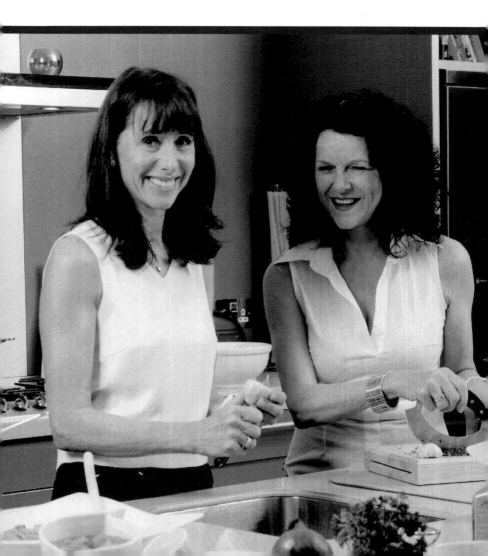

Once you become a *soupaholic* you never look back. You lose unwanted pounds and keep them off, you have more energy and take on new challenges, you become more tolerant and less stressed, you body swerve colds and viruses, your skin, hair and nails improve and digestive issues become a thing of the past.

Bold claims perhaps but as you read on you will begin to understand why soup can be your very best friend. And, talking of best friends, I can only make these bold claims and pass on my soup words of wisdom thanks to **my** best friend, Jean Barr who has not only devised all the soup recipes in this book but over the many years I have been helping people to get lean, stay lean and feel great has somehow managed to concoct soups to accommodate every taste and preference - a rare talent!

But before I launch into why and how soup works on so many levels let me give you a little background on me and Jean and why we decided not only to write **Soup Can Make You Thin** but also to set up our complementary website, www.souperydupery.com.

We have been friends for over 25 years, having met when we both worked in the recruitment industry and aside from the fact that we both share a pocky Scottish sense of humour which enables us to laugh, often hysterically at ourselves and generally cope with whatever life slings at us, our shared love of food is a major player in our friendship. We both passionately believe that a fit, lean body can only be achieved and maintained when your daily diet includes deliciously tasty food and a generous helping of your favourites - **bean sprouts may be a great addition to a fat loss plan but not every day thanks!** So, I am the one who spends most of my waking hours keeping up to speed with nutritional science, scribbling articles and books on the subject and devising diets for fat loss and better health and Jean is the one who shops, chops, slices, dices and creates fabulous soups to meet my often exacting remit. Then, we both dig in, tweak the recipes and dig in again!

One of the questions we are regularly asked, usually by fellow diners is how we both manage to stay so slim and yet eat so much? Many assume that we just got lucky, have 'slim' genes and have never had a weight problem but that is far from the truth. Both of us struggled with our weight for many years (and yes, we have photos to prove it!), both of us tried every new fad diet that hit the bookshelves and both of us embraced all sorts of daft and sometimes health-threatening tactics such as diet pills, herbal concoctions, fasting and the rest before it finally dawned on us that **eating more not less** might be the answer and it was. But, more of what? Soup of course!

There are a host of biochemical reasons behind **why** soup can make you thin and whilst I intend to cover them all, it will be brief. Not because they are unimportant - far from it and many readers may be keen to understand and perhaps further investigate the nutritional principles outlined. For this reason, I have included a list of references at the back of the book.

The reason for biochemical brevity is because, in my view we are bombarded with way too much advice on **why** we should eat this and not that and not nearly enough simple, straightforward advice on **how to bring it all together and put it into practice** in what for most of us is a busy life. Countless dieters I have worked with over the years have asked me to keep the science to a minimum and just tell them what to do. They want to get slim, stay slim, know they are getting a wealth of essential nutrients but simply can't spare the time to get to grips with the nutritional pros and cons before launching into a new eating programme. As one rather direct client once said to me; "That's your job". Point taken! So I am asking you to trust that I have done the groundwork and am going to tell you **a little about why soup can make you thin and a lot about how to ensure it does.**

Soups to Suit **You**

This is not a book weighed down with rigid rules and all soup suggestions are nutritious and health-enhancing. However, permanent fat loss is a great deal more likely when we see rapid results in the early stages and many dieters find it easier when there is a plan to follow. Others find a plan much too restrictive and demanding so prefer to devise their own. We have endeavoured to cover all tastes and lifestyles and in doing so have split our soup recipes into three categories as follows:

SuperSkinny Soups

To make and choose when you are looking to shed fat fast.

Skinny Soups

To make and choose when you are close to your goal or have decided to shed the pounds at a more leisurely pace.

FatBustForever Soups

To make and choose when you are close to or have reached your goal and want to maintain your new lean, healthy body.

This book doesn't include pictures of our soups but you can see them all on our website, www.souperydupery.com. Some of the shots are fabulous thanks to the awesome photographic skills of Keny Drew, www.kenydrew. co.uk but others are our own feeble attempts. Clearly, our photographic skills are not in the same league as our soup skills but with luck they will give you some idea of how colourful, tasty and full of goodness the soups are! You can also sign up to become a *soupaholic*, giving you access to all the latest soup news, reviews, recipes and general soupy gossip.

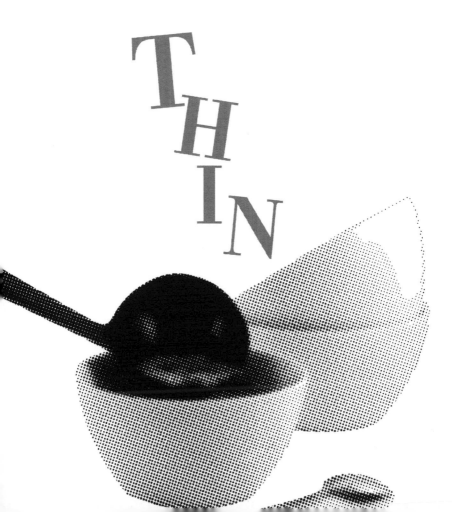

WHY SOUP CAN MAKE YOU THIN

Some of the points below have proven research behind them and you will find the relevant studies quoted at the back of the book. Some are gaining ground on the nutritional science platform thanks to the dedication of the relatively few in global terms who work tirelessly to increase our awareness of the importance of good nutrition for a good and healthy life and trust me, these people risk a lot when they post their findings as 'the establishment' is often quick to criticise. Others are based on my personal experience and the experience of others in my field who have helped countless numbers of people to finally lose the flab and find a route to better health. If you want a lean, fit body there are many ways to achieve it and whilst proven science has a major influence, it is not the only way.

Soup is a Liquid Meal with a Difference

The hormone, ghrelin which is released by specific cells in the stomach wall is one of the major players in the body's appetite system. When the stomach is empty, ghrelin ferries the message to the brain telling us we are hungry, but when the stomach wall is stretched the cells stop producing ghrelin and the appetite signal is turned off so the longer the stomach remains full the longer we feel satisfied and the less likely we are to overeat. Soup has been shown to keep the stomach wall stretched for up to an hour and a half longer than the same food taken with water because the blend of food and water is digested differently from the solid food plus water. In one study researchers asked women to eat chicken casserole on its own, chicken casserole with a glass of water or chicken casserole with the same amount of water added to make a soup. They were then allowed to eat whatever they liked for lunch. Those who ate the soup consumed around 100kcals fewer. In another study carried out by the same researchers, when adults received a bowl of low-calorie vegetable soup 15 minutes before a pasta lunch, they consumed 20 percent fewer calories in the complete meal. The BBC did a similar experiment as part of a documentary which achieved comparable results.

Soup Satisfies Hunger

Another appetite hormone, leptin can be a major adversary if not carefully managed. Leptin is produced by the fat cells and tells the brain when energy stores are replenished and we have had enough to eat. When this hormone is working optimally we are better able to control when we eat and how much we eat but it is easily disrupted and if the signals to the brain are scrambled it is all too easy to just go along with our desires resulting in us gorging rather than grazing and likely weight gain. When the communication lines are open we eat when we are hungry and we stop when we are full but leptin can get caught up in a kind of *biochemical traffic jam*. The fullness message doesn't get through and the brain continues to tell us that we are hungry so we keep looking for further nourishment until we are satisfied. This is nothing short of a disaster when we are trying to lose weight. **Leptin sensitivity**, where the messages are a bit fuzzy and erratic is on the increase and numerous surveys show that diets overloaded with sugary, starchy foods and light on energy-dense and nourishing foods are largely to blame. And to make matters worse, over time **leptin resistance** can develop, where the brain neither receives nor responds to the messages. Our hormonal system thrives on balance and leptin can only play its important role in appetite management when the system is regularly provided with top grade fuel - carbohydrates, protein, fats, vitamins, minerals and water are the six essentials in a top grade fuel. A great bowl of soup has the lot.

Thick Soup or Thin Soup?

One study tested how much the participants ate for lunch once a week for five weeks after consuming 'soup four ways' prior to their main dish; broth and vegetables served separately, chunky vegetable soup, chunky pureed vegetable soup and pureed vegetable soup. Results showed that consuming the soup significantly reduced test meal intake and total meal energy intake compared to having no soup by an average of 26 percent. The type of soup had no significant effect which indicates that you can pretty much suit yourself, which is good news for *soupaholics* everywhere - we all have preferences. It is worth noting however, that there is substantial evidence that we generally eat less of a chunky soup and feel full more quickly which is an added bonus when fat loss is the goal. Many of our recipes can be adapted to produce your preferred consistency.

Soup Fights Water Retention

Retaining fluid within the body is not just a nuisance when it comes to how uncomfortable our clothes feel; over time it also presents health risks (high blood pressure, type 2 diabetes, kidney problems). The first piece of advice is usually to increase water consumption. Many find this confusing as the *more equals less* idea seems somewhat contradictory, but retention basically means fluid is being **held** within body cells rather that **entering and leaving** on a regular basis to assist in almost every biochemical reaction that takes place. If you don't give your body water, it holds on to water so it won't run out. The liquid in soup and the water content of most vegetables provide good levels in every bowl.

Another reason water retention occurs is when there is too much sodium in our diet and not enough potassium. These minerals need to be in balance to allow the transport of nutrients into and waste out of the body cells. An imbalance of these minerals is very common, principally because there is too much salt in many diets; not just the stuff we add to our food but the crazy levels present in many processed and fast foods and most junk foods (more about salt later). Apart from cutting back on salt we need to increase our levels of potassium to get the balance back. Vegetables offer good levels of potassium and soups invariably include a good selection of vegetables.

Finally, protein is important. When there is insufficient protein in our diet, fluid is retained to protect what protein we have from being broken down and used to keep the *repairing and rebuilding* network operating. Muscles are a particularly rich source of body protein so they are usually targeted first. Most of us are all too familiar with the disturbing pictures of starving children in countries where famine is common. Woefully thin arms and legs, protruding bones and swollen bellies are the norm as their little bodies struggle to hang onto life. Soup offers an excellent opportunity to ensure that we get good levels of protein in our daily diet. Where our soups are predominantly vegetable-based, we always recommend a protein topping or a protein snack alongside (see *Protein Extras* in the recipe section).

Soup is Damned Near Nutritional Perfection

If you get the mix right! When you are trying to lose weight it is easy to become obsessed about how to achieve the perfect balance of essential nutrients and there's no shortage of conflicting advice on what constitutes a balanced, fat fighting diet! So let me clarify a few important points in the next chapter.

NUTRITIONAL
PERFECTION IN A

B
O
W
L

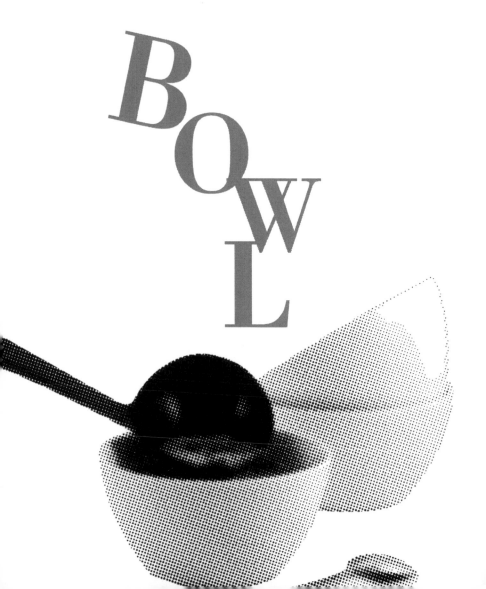

Carbohydrates Are Monumentally Confusing!

Carbohydrate foods are vital because they provide the raw materials that enable the body cells to create energy but which carbohydrates we need and how much presents possibly the greatest confusion for dieters. They are often split into two categories; **simple carbohydrates** which are broken down and release their sugars quickly, don't keep us energised for long, are generally lacking in nutritional greatness and should be limited and **complex carbohydrates** which are broken down more slowly, keep us energised for longer, are richer in nutritional goodness and should be consumed regularly. However, it is not quite that simple and in my view, and I am certainly not alone here, this somewhat simplistic advice is one of the major reasons global waistlines are increasing at an alarming rate.

Which foods do most people crave? Carbohydrate-rich foods. Bingeing on foods that are high in protein and fat is hard; most people can't do it. When we are faced with a plate piled high with large, fat, juicy steaks we may manage one, maybe two but generally we feel full fairly quickly. Sadly, the same doesn't apply when it comes to starchy and sugary carbohydrates. We can eat fries, crisps, popcorn, biscuits, cakes and hot buttered toast until the cows come home and still manage just one more helping. Why is this? Why does the appetite switch that tells us we can't eat any more steak not tell us that we shouldn't cram in another slice of pizza?

One overfeeding experiment saw a group of people eating a whopping 10,000kcals of predominantly starchy, sugary carbohydrate foods and yet they were still hungry later in the day whereas the other group who were faced with 'plates of pork chops a mile high' couldn't consume anywhere near the same number of calories. Researchers discovered that both the anticipation of the starchy, sugary foods and the actual eating of them caused the secretion of insulin (the fat storing hormone) in the first group. Not only in larger amounts than the other group but more regularly. Interestingly, other experiments show that people who are seriously overweight or clinically obese often opt for sugary, starchy foods when hunger strikes.

A thousand calories of popcorn is easy, a thousand calories of steak is a struggle!

Where the confusion lies for many trying to shed the flab is that much of the advice we are bombarded with involves overly-complicated explanations of why repeated secretion of insulin into the bloodstream to keep levels of glucose within safe limits leads to fat storage. Starchy, sugary carbohydrates satisfy our need for glucose to create energy fast when we are hungry, stressed, overtired etc. but they come at a price. They don't sustain us for long and they don't supply us with the level of micronutrients (vitamins, minerals and accessory nutrients) required to assist in the creation of energy by the trillions of body cells that are endeavouring to keep us firing on all cylinders. Hunger strikes all too quickly and the brain tells us to eat. When we reach for more of the same the process starts all over again and whilst we feel full and satisfied for a short time, it doesn't last long.

If we want to burn fat for energy in a bid to get the fat cells to shrink and stay shrunk, we have to respond to hunger with foods that not only provide nourishment but also keep us feeling fuller for longer, don't overwork the pancreas which is put in the unenviable position of having to keep producing insulin to ensure that blood sugar levels remain neither too high nor too low and don't ask too much of the body cells which, when continually asked to *open the gates* to let yet more glucose in can all-too-easily become a little lacklustre.

It is not just the continued eating of starchy, sugary carbohydrates that makes demands on the pancreas to secrete insulin, it's also the anticipation of these foods that can lead to low levels of sugar in the bloodstream and create the very real need for balance with yet more sugar. This is dangerous for dieters, particularly if they are tempted to follow very low calorie programmes or cut back on certain food groups. The importance of getting a good balance of the *Big 6* (carbohydrates, protein, fats, vitamins, minerals and water) at regular intervals throughout the day cannot be over-emphasised.

So, how do we feed the body cells rather than deprive them or confuse them?

- **Give them fuel** with energy-dense carbohydrates.

- **Eat protein with every meal and snack** to slow down the release of glucose into the bloodstream and moderate the secretion of the fat-storing hormone, insulin.
- **Add essential fats** to make us feel fuller for longer, keep hunger at bay and further moderate the insulin release.
- **Enrich them** with foods packed with vitamins and minerals to feed the enzymes that play such an important role in efficient energy production.

Top Notch Starches

Great carbohydrates are carbohydrates that feed our energy requirements without creating the need for more all too soon and those that tick the box and are included in our soups are:

- Root Vegetables
- Beans
- Lentils
- Chickpeas
- Broad beans and peas
- Brown rice
- Brown basmati rice
- Oats
- Barley

This point is crucial for both short term fat loss and lasting fat loss.

The body is essentially a carbohydrate/glucose/fat-storing environment and whilst we don't advocate the absence of carbohydrates or very low carbohydrate diets, we see no point whatsoever in allowing starch-rich carbohydrates to fill half a plateful of food or the bulk of a bowl of soup. They are important, they are essential and they keep us fuelled but they are part of a team and the other players deserve equal standing and respect.

Protein Packs a Punch

One of the rationales for eating a diet relatively rich in protein is that this macronutrient, calorie-for-calorie sates the appetite most effectively. Individuals who adopt this type of diet almost always eat less; often, several hundred calories less per day. This is believed to be because better blood sugar stability is achieved which helps guard against episodes of low blood sugar which triggers false hunger and food cravings - usually for starchy and sugary carbohydrates. There are also studies that indicate that higher protein diets may assist weight loss through increased thermogenesis. After eating, our metabolism generally enjoys a boost, rather like what happens when we put fuel on a fire. The thermogenic effect of protein is greater than the thermogenic effect of carbohydrates or fats and lasts longer. It is not huge, but over time can have quite a marked effect.

Protein may only account for about 12 percent of our total body weight but that 12 percent defines us as living, breathing, standing, moving, thinking and functioning human beings. Proteins are the building blocks of our uniqueness. They are present in every cell and are the chief components of skin, bones, hair, nails, muscles and hormones. They also protect us from disease by creating antibodies that fight foreign invaders and transport oxygen from the lungs to body cells to create energy from food. But, what makes us truly unique is our DNA and every cell uses the information encoded in our genes, which is a kind of *protein library* as the blueprint for making the hundreds of thousands of different proteins that give us our uniqueness.

We don't store protein to the same extent we do carbohydrates and fats so we must include them regularly in our diet to ensure that we have sufficient levels to achieve all of the above, so little and often is where it's at. Whilst we don't intend to include a chapter outlining how significant regular exercise is in any fat loss plan, it makes a massive difference to how we look, how we feel and how much energy we have. Muscle tissue is active tissue and requires a lot of energy from food plus good levels of protein in our diet allows for muscle growth and repair. Muscle is also denser than body fat so **takes up less room pound for pound** so if you lose two pounds of fat whilst gaining two pounds of muscle your body weight won't change but your body shape will - for the better. So what you actually weigh is in some instances immaterial; more about why you should bin the scales and instead, use our Waistband Method later. Professional sportsmen and women, soldiers in the armed forces, bodybuilders etc. who have lots of muscle and very little body fat often weigh a great deal more than their *couch potato* counterparts but their bodies look fitter and healthier despite the fact that their weight puts many of them in the overweight category if their BMI is used as a benchmark.

Many of our soups include good levels of protein and where they don't, we always recommend you add a topping or a snack on the side (see *Protein Extras* in the recipe section) to ensure you stay in the 'little, often and fast fat burning' lane.

And What About Fat?

Weight loss is about fat loss and not necessarily about consuming less calories. There was a time, around twenty years ago when fats were everything that was deemed bad from a health perspective and the WHO (World Health Organisation) decreed that we should give them a very wide berth. How things change on the nutritional stage! The emerging greatness of essential fats (Omega 3 fats in particular) is **so big** that understanding their role in improving all-round health and perhaps even curbing the global obesity crises could well take centre stage in the near future.

Around 60 percent of the brain is fat and without it communication of thoughts, feelings and reactions as well as our interpretation and sense of everything around us is impaired. Fat also ensures hormones stay in prime condition, particularly sex hormones. Fat is truly our friend and ally for energy, fitness, fat loss, heart health, immunity, procreation and longevity. But which fats should we eat?

It is a complicated subject but in an effort to cut through the confusion, we can split the foods rich in fats into four camps:

- Those that **must** be included in our diet because we can't make them within the body and are essential for the above functions.
- Those that are **not essential** for the above functions but offer other health benefits.

- Those that **we don't need** to include in our diet because we can make them within the body but when eaten in small quantities offer health benefits.
- Those that **should be avoided** as they do us no favours health-wise.

Group one includes most seeds and nuts and their oils and butters, oily fish, soya beans and tofu, group two includes olives, avocados, peanuts and their oil, beans, lentils, chickpeas, eggs and some green vegetables and group three includes lean meat, poultry, game and low fat dairy products. Group four is the real danger zone. Trans fats, hydrogenated fats and semi-hydrogenated fats are fats that started out as health-giving oils derived from plants but have been altered and subjected to a dizzying array of chemical and heat processes to manufacture them more cheaply and give them and products containing them a longer shelf life. They offer little nutritional benefit to the body and when consumed regularly interfere with the metabolism of the fats in the other three groups, reducing their effectiveness and increasing the risk of inflammation within the body which can, over time compromise health. Sadly, these altered fats give foods the kind of *fatty* taste that makes us want to eat more of them and are present in many processed and fast foods and most junk foods. The good news is that they have to be itemised on the food label so look out for them and avoid them where possible. Most of the vegetable oils bottled in clear plastic containers that line supermarket shelves should also be viewed with suspicion; the fact that they are being sold at knock-down prices is usually an indication that they have been over-processed and contain few if any health-giving fats. Instead, use olive, rapeseed, avocado and coconut oil for cooking and use nut and seed oils for drizzling over soups, vegetables and salads and adding to smoothies.

What's the Scoop on Salt?

Consider this:

- Around 10 percent of our daily consumption of salt is inherent in food.
- Around 5-10 percent of our daily sodium intake comes from salt added to fresh foods during cooking. And, even if we add salt at the table, this makes up only around 6 percent of our daily intake.

- **But, estimates reveal that over 70 percent of our daily salt intake comes from processed, pre-packaged, and prepared foods**. Why? Because it is a fabulous preserver (of food, not life!) and hugely increases shelf life.

If you eat only unprocessed foods; fruits, vegetables, whole grains, nuts, seeds, seafood, red meats, poultry, game, eggs, dairy produce that you prepare yourself with a light hand on the salt shaker you take in far more potassium than sodium (not to mention all the vitamins, minerals, fibre, phytonutrients and healthy fats involved) and more potassium than sodium is the way to go.

There are now many table salts available which have around 60 percent less sodium than ordinary table salt and are enriched with magnesium and potassium to create a good balance of these three minerals. *Solo Salt, Pan Salt* and *Smart Salt* are good examples but there are others - seek them out.

A number of studies show a marked improvement in blood pressure among those who make the switch from high sodium salt to low sodium and high magnesium/potassium salt and whilst the cynic in me has to point out that like many studies, some were funded by companies who are likely to benefit from increased sales on the back of these positive results, there is little argument that reducing sodium levels and increasing magnesium and potassium levels through our food choices is going to reduce the risks and improve our health.

This leads us nicely onto the use of stock cubes, stock gels and pastes and ready-made stocks in soup recipes. Some get better press than others on the sodium front and global awareness of *too much salt in our diet* has prompted/forced many manufacturers to greatly reduce the amount of salt in their products which is very good news. However, **and this is important**; some stock cubes may contain as much as half the recommended daily intake of sodium but most recipes where stock is required use just one or two cubes and make four to six servings. So, even if you were to make a pot and have a bowl of the same soup four times in one day you would still be below the danger line and consuming less than you would if you opted for a large takeaway pizza, many of which contain more than the whole recommended daily intake and from a nutritional point of view will never compete with four bowls of good, nourishing soup.

Salting your soup:

- Don't *double salt*. If you use stock cubes/gels in the cooking, don't add salt either later in the process or at the table.

- If you are making your own stocks, taste, taste and taste again to ensure they are flavoursome and add a little salt at the end before using, refrigerating or freezing.

- Where we recommend the addition of salt in the cooking, use low sodium, magnesium/potassium-rich salt or sea salt wherever possible.

- Get into the habit of using herbs and spices, a splash of vinegar or soy sauce or *Herbamare* (a mix of sea salt and dried herbs) to add flavour before serving your soups.

- If you are buying soups off the shelf, steer clear of those that say 'low fat' or 'low calorie' on the label - salt is often added to give them flavour.

- Look at the label: where it says *Salt or Salt Equivalent*, 1.5g per 100g is high, 0.3g is low. **Aim for a maximum of 0.6g**. Where is says *Sodium*, 0.5g per 100g is high, 0.1g is low. **Aim for a maximum of 0.2g**.

Interestingly, there is some evidence that we can't easily tell the difference in salt levels in food. In a number of trials at Harvard Medical School reductions of as much as 25 percent remained undetected by the volunteers so try and get used to using less salt over the space of a couple of weeks, savour the flavours of the ingredients and see how your need for salt might be blunted.

Calories, Bathroom Scales and The Waistband Method

We don't like counting, particularly calories. Some dieters pride themselves on being able to rattle off the calorie count of loads of foods and drinks and/ or have apps on their phones which do super-quick calculations but little of it makes sense. A good-sized bowl of our *Lamb and Bean Soup* probably has a calorie count of around 140kcals but is bursting with fat busting and filling beans, quality lean protein, healthy fats, nutritious vegetables and of course water. It provides **quality** ingredients, a **quality** balance of nutrients and **quality** calories. A standard can of cola provides around the same number of calories but offers little more than sugar. Many experts agree that the various calorie myths; 'a calorie is a calorie', 'eat less exercise more', 'to lose one pound of fat we should consume 500kcals less per day' etc. are largely responsible for the current obesity crisis. And, the countless years where low fat/high starch diets were championed haven't helped! Certainly, if we regularly consume more than we need to fulfil our energy requirements we will, over time gain weight just as if we regularly take in less than we need we will lose weight. But the body is much more sophisticated than that, requires a great deal of energy to stay in good working order and will use every trick in the book to hang onto stored energy if it is under threat. Too few or too many calories or a diet loaded with **poor quality calories** pose a threat and the quickest and easiest way to preserve energy is for the body to turn down the metabolic rate. This is nothing short of a disaster when we want to shed fat and lose inches and the only way to avoid this metabolic meltdown is to feed the body regularly with **top quality calories** that not only demand the body uses lots of energy to process them but also provide us with the essential nutrients to keep the metabolic fire burning brightly.

We don't like counting pounds either (other than for cooking purposes). **Weighing scales should be a kitchen essential, not a bathroom accessory.** Most of us know when we are overweight, we don't need a set of scales to confirm it. Our clothes become a bit tight or we have to buy a bigger size and we don't like what we see in the mirror. Fat has accumulated on our hips, thighs, bellies and bums and this is what we want to shift. A lean, fit body is a body with a low fat percentage (14 to 17 percent in men, 21 to 24 percent in women) and those who achieve this goal sometimes tip the scales at more than the recommended weight for their height, body type and age but they look and feel great. Also, our weight fluctuates, sometimes fairly drastically for a myriad of reasons. Dieters who are obsessed with weighing themselves every morning quickly become disheartened when the scales show no loss or worse still a gain, their day doesn't get off to a good start and they begin to question the diet they are slavishly following. What also occurs in some cases is that the no

HOW TO

FIT SOUP INTO YOUR

DAY

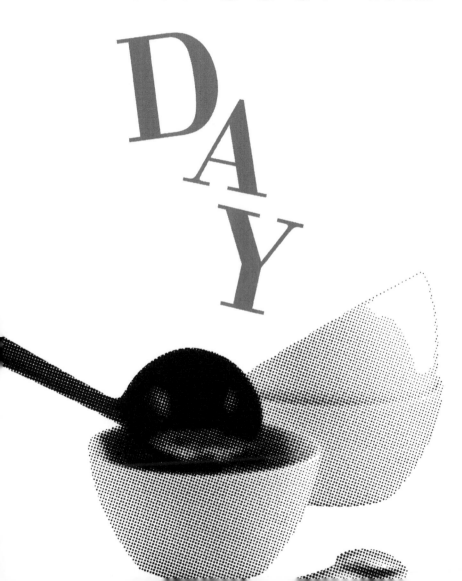

Now you have decided to become a *soupaholic* you might want to decide which category you best fit into:

- You like cooking and you want your soups to be as fresh as possible so you are happy to spend time shopping for ingredients and make all your own soups.
- You like cooking and you want your soups to be as fresh as possible but time is often the enemy.
- You rarely find time to cook but are willing to set aside a couple of hours a week to make a batch or two and freeze in manageable portions.
- You never cook other than heating up foods in the microwave or on the hob but are willing to 'have a go'.
- You can't cook and the prospect of making soup fills you with terror.
- You rarely eat in and need help to decide which soups to select when you are out and about.

Whilst we urge you, whatever category you fall into to get the apron on and the blender out, we appreciate that for some this may not be feasible or achievable so for that reason we have included some advice on 'best and worst choice soups' available from the chiller cabinet, the supermarket shelves, high street chains or when you are lunching or dining out in the recipe section. Soup producers, from the biggest factories to the smallest restaurants and everyone in between add new and seasonal varieties almost daily so keep an eye on our website, www.souperydoupery.com, where we will endeavour to keep you up to speed with what's on offer - well I will, Jean is a hard nut to crack when it comes to anything other than home-made soups!

Soup for Breakfast
(or as soon as food fits into your early morning schedule)

Try it for three or four days in just one week and see what happens. It is likely that some or all of the following occur:

- **You won't need your regular early morning cup of tea/coffee.**
- **You won't be hungry mid morning and struggle to resist a sugary snack.**
- **You won't experience the same energy dips you are used to after a cereal/toast breakfast.**
- **You won't count the hours until lunchtime.**

Have a mug or bowl of **any** of our soups (**SuperSkinny Soups** if you are looking to shed fat fast, **Skinny Soups** if you are taking a more leisurely approach, **Fat Bust Forever Soups** if you are close to or have reached your goal). There will be some soups that don't appeal at this time of day so pick the ones you like best - you don't need an additional challenge first thing in the morning! As you get comfortable with the notion and practice of slurping soup for breakfast a few times a week you can get a bit more adventurous; experiment and find what works for you.

On a personal note:
Neither Jean nor I would thank you for a big bowl of cereal first thing in the morning. We both have busy work schedules and the same domestic commitments most of us have to deal with but as mentioned, we both like food (a lot!) and hate being hungry so when the day ahead is likely to be demanding we want something filling and full of flavour early doors and frankly, a bowl of cereal just doesn't cut it. Where's the protein, where are the essential and filling fats, where's the satisfaction, where's the deliciousness? Yes, there is fibre if you pick the best possible mix of cereals, yes there are some essential nutrients if you don't focus on the overly-processed varieties but in our view, that's about it. No thanks, not for us. We do have other favourite breakfasts and early morning choices (see *Non-Soup Breakfasts and Early Morning Choices* in the recipe section) but soup can't be beaten for good all round nourishment at least three times a week. However, like many whose lives are a constant rush we don't always manage to fit breakfast into our day but that's not a major nourishment issue - we both favour a big handbag and there's always something lurking in there that will keep us going until mid morning or lunchtime (see *Non-Soup Super Quick Snacks* in the recipe section)!

Soup Mid Morning and/or Mid Afternoon

(This works on **so** many levels)

There are as many nutritional experts that champion having snacks and small meals five or six times a day for successful long term fat loss as there are those who propose that three good meals a day with no snacks is the route. So, who do you believe? Yourself! We are all different and what works for one person is not necessarily the solution for another.

Food is fuel but how much we need and how often is dependent on our biochemistry, our health status and our lifestyle. If you are the type who thrives on three good meals a day and don't suffer from energy dips in between then that's what you should stick to most days. If you are the type that can't get through to lunch or dinner without something nourishing mid morning and/or mid afternoon then clearly, small and often is the route for you. There are no hard and fast rules. Plus, there can be days where energy requirements are greater than others which has a lot to do with hormone balance which is never easy, particularly for women.

To date, over fifty hormones have been identified in the human body but the ones that have the greatest influence on how successfully we bust fat forever are:

- **The thyroid hormones:** T3 and thyroxine.
- **The stress hormones:** adrenaline and cortisol.
- **The sex hormones:** oestrogen, progesterone and testosterone.
- **The blood glucose hormones:** insulin and glucagon.
- **The hunger and appetite hormones:** ghrelin and leptin.

If any of these are either under or over-performing they affect how the others behave.

Our eating and exercising habits, the amount of physical, emotional, nutritional and environmental stress we are under, our age and health history, the interplay of our sex hormones and a host of other contributory factors have a direct impact on how they all perform. Where fat loss is the goal, the ones we need to concentrate on in the early stages are the hunger and appetite hormones, ghrelin and leptin which have already been discussed. We want to achieve a situation where we only eat when we are hungry and stop eating when we are full but that's a lot easier in theory than it is in practice. In my experience of working with umpteen dieters who have lost weight for good, small and often has been the winner and soup snacks have played a major part in their success.

A good strategy is to take a little time to uncover the times of the day when energy dips occur. For some it is mid morning and/or mid afternoon for others it is late evening and for many it is around 6pm when the day has been manic and the urge to scarf down whatever comes to hand is overwhelming. It very much depends on how much is being demanded of your body at any given time but once you begin to recognise the signs of a looming energy dip you can confront it before it has a chance to cause a major diversion. We have included a list of nutritionally-balanced, convenient and easy to throw-together snacks (see *Non-Soup Super Quick Snacks* in the recipe section) but we continue to champion a mug or small bowl of soup as the snack of choice to keep the hunger and appetite hormones happy, particularly if you haven't had time to *break your fast* early in the day.

Soup at Lunchtime
(or as a major part of your lunch)

This is the **very best time of day** to have a cracking big bowl of filling soup with all the trimmings. For good health, weight management and day-long energy many in the wonderful world of nutrition recommend that we should 'breakfast like a king, lunch like a lord and dine like a pauper' and yes it makes some nutritional sense but many of us have to rush breakfast, grab breakfast on the way to work or don't find time for breakfast at all and the early to mid morning snack is the only thing that keeps us going until lunchtime. Equally, dinner is often the only time of day when we get a chance to stop the clock and sit down to a decent meal. But, a big meal late in the day can be a waistline expander, particularly if we then hit the couch to watch TV or sit for hours at the computer checking out what our Facebook friends are up to. We suggest that lunch should be elevated to altogether greater heights and given regal status. So, here's what we suggest:

- **Breakfast when you can.**
- **Make lunch a priority.**
- **Dine cleverly and carefully.**
- **Snack to prevent energy crashes.**

The reason soup features as a great lunchtime option in almost every fat loss plan I have devised over many years is principally because the middle of the day is the time to include a few starchy carbohydrates which fill you up and provide much-needed energy to get you through the afternoon and early evening. The brain is glucose-greedy and if the sugars from carbohydrate foods are in short supply (as in very low carbohydrate diets) you know about it all too quickly; loss of concentration, irritability, cravings for a sugary snack or a desperate need to put your head down for ten minutes. However, not all starchy carbohydrates are created equal so as mentioned you should concentrate on the **top notch starches** and only include the others occasionally if choice is limited or when you have reached your fat loss goal.

Soup Early Evening
(when temptation threatens)

I promised I was going to keep the science to a minimum and have already discussed how difficult it can be to keep the major hormones in balance. If you don't struggle to fight temptation at this time of the day you are very, very lucky but you are in the minority. This can be a huge obstacle when we are trying to lose weight; I have lost count of the number of emails I have received from dieters who have stuck rigidly to my recommendations during the day but fall apart and hit the alcohol/salty snacks/childrens' leftovers and the rest when the day has been demanding. At the risk of repeating myself, hormones are usually to blame but here it is more likely to be the stress hormones which are causing problems. Cortisol in particular. Cortisol is the hormone that tells the body to **increase the appetite and store fat** when stress is ongoing. This was a life-saver for our ancestors when the major stresses they encountered were either fighting for survival or having to deal with days or weeks on end where food was scarce. Stored fat meant they could live to fight another day. Today's stressors are very different but the body's reaction is still the same. A day swamped with deadlines, worries, time issues, lack of nutrients and a whole host of other kinds of stress prompt the continued release of this irritatingly-efficient hormone and without a good helping of discipline and willpower it can be very difficult to quell its enthusiasm but a soup snack can work miracles.

Soup As Your Evening Meal
(or as part of your evening meal)

Whether you opt for soup in the evening or not is totally up to you. Soup can either **be** your evening meal if you have eaten well and regularly throughout the day and are not overly hungry, can form **part of your evening meal** if you are hungry or **can be ignored** in favour of other dishes. If you have already completed the *10 Day Flab-Fighting Soup Diet* but are still looking to shed more pounds, go for the **SuperSkinny** or the **Skinny** soup recommendations. If you have reached your fat loss goal select any of the soups. There is just one proviso and that is unless you exercise in the evening or have a physically-demanding night ahead, **avoid starchy carbohydrates at this time of the day**. Occasionally is fine, if you are out and the choice is limited they won't do much harm and if you have reached your fat loss goal they are unlikely to cause weight gain unless they become a nightly feature. So, if you are having soup, concentrate on the suggestions that don't include starches and if you are having a 'knife and fork meal' fill half the plate with vegetables or salad, have a decent portion of protein (fish, shellfish, poultry, red meat, tofu, eggs, low fat dairy products) and use nuts, seeds, nut and seed oils and avocado as additions/garnishes to ensure you get a good helping of fat busting essential fats.

Soup After Exercise
(if you exercise in the evening)

Dependent on what you have eaten during the day, there are days when a good bout of exercise can leave you absolutely starving afterwards. Once you have used up the readily-available glucose for any kind of physically-demanding session, your body calls on the stored glucose (glycogen) in your liver and muscles to keep providing energy. When you finish, the fat cells are called upon to release their energy to replenish stores - that's when the fat burning commences and if you are trying to shed the flab that's exactly what you want. However, what you eat post-exercise (particularly later in the day) is critical to both continued refuelling and to the recovery and repair of muscles so you can continue with your regular training programme the next day. The first nutritional priority is to replace any fluid lost during exercise but research also shows that combining carbohydrate with protein within 30 minutes of exercise results in more stored glycogen; the optimal recommended ratio is 4:1. There are, of course many ways to achieve this desired combination of water, carbohydrate and protein but it's hard to beat soup. It's warming, comforting, tasty, easy on the digestive system, hydrating, bursting with antioxidants to minimise muscle damage and most of our soups that include starches deliver something pretty close to the recommended carbohydrate to protein ratio.

Soup Before Bed
(if you have trouble sleeping)

An entire (and rather large) book could be written on how, when and what to eat and drink to get more and better sleep. Lack of sleep plagues us all occasionally and many suffer nightly. However, for the purposes of this book I am going to concentrate on serotonin, a chemical that is produced in the brain and when levels are good, encourages feelings of calm which help promote sleep. Our serotonin levels are influenced by the amount of tryptophan (an essential amino acid found in protein foods) in the blood and as blood and brain levels of tryptophan rise and fall, so do levels of serotonin. Tryptophan can be the runt of the litter when it comes to competing with the other amino acids to get from the bloodstream into the brain but a little carbohydrate added to a protein-rich snack creates a diversion allowing tryptophan to take the stage. Foods rich in tryptophan include turkey, chicken, tofu, spinach, asparagus and bok choy. Our bedtime *Turkey/Tofu & Spinach Soup* includes some of these plus a little carbohydrate to assist in the transport. Whilst we generally discourage starchy carbohydrates after 6pm for the reasons mentioned, this is one exception. There are no guarantees but it is certainly worth a try if you find it difficult to get to sleep. It is also a good strategy if you regularly wake up in the very early hours of the morning and can't get back to sleep. This is often as a result of low blood sugar and a bedtime soup snack can help to avoid this.

Soup On The Go
(or when time is tight)

Fresh, homemade soups are tops. You know exactly what is going into them and you can gauge the salt content. With a bit of planning you can ensure that you have soup portions in the freezer which can be quickly defrosted and reheated but there are always occasions when this is simply not practical. This is where ready-made soups come in and the choice is vast. So which should you pick when time is tight or you are out and about and you are watching your waistline? A common theme has been predominating over the last few years with regard to how much salt is in ready-made soups with all the usual health warnings that go along with the territory. One recent survey compared the amount of salt in fifteen different bowls of minestrone; some were canned, cartoned or bagged, others were from fast food outlets and a couple were restaurant fare. They ranged from just 1.2g to a whopping 4g. Salt has already been discussed and if you regularly opt for soups made by someone other than yourself, you **do** have to keep an eye on the numbers. Follow the guidelines in 'Salting Your Soup' if there is a label or ask if there isn't. You won't always get an answer sadly, but it's important to remember that a good soup has a lot going for it nutritionally and even those with a little too much salt are generally going to be a better choice than a vast number of ready snacks and meals on offer.

We regularly taste and test on-the-go soups and plan to give you our views through our website and in our newsletters but for now, here are a few pointers:

- Go for protein-based soups; meat, poultry, game, fish, shellfish, tofu, beans, lentils, peas, chickpeas.
- If it's a predominantly vegetable soup top it with some cooked meat, poultry, fish, shellfish, tofu or have some protein on the side.
- Avoid the ones that are super-thick with pasta, rice or potatoes.

- Avoid the creamy ones unless it's coconut milk or coconut cream.
- If it's a supermarket soup, go for the ones with the shortest shelf life; they are likely to have less salt and fewer preservatives.
- Check the ingredients on the label where possible and if it's full of *emulsifiers, regulators, starches, syrups* and *extracts*, give it a wide berth.

We have included a list of best and worst on-the-go soup choices in the recipe section but a great tactic is to *Google* your favourites and check both the ingredients and the fat, sugar and salt levels - they often surprise. For example: we recently had two soups from a well-known-for-freshness chain. Both were delicious. One might expect the *Ham, Lentil and Chunky Vegetable* to have more sugar, saturated fat and salt than the *Spiced Tomato* but no. The *Spiced Tomato* had more of all three - it pays to check!

Very quick soup snacks (cuppa soups etc.) don't have a lot going for them. It's hard to find **any** that don't include unrecognisable and unpronounceable ingredients and those that have words like *slim, healthy* or *low* on the front are often the worst offenders. When manufacturers vastly reduce the calories in a product, they have to add the above-mentioned enhancers to give the product some taste! The more *real* food words on the label the better.

Miso soup is readily available in sachets and pastes and some high street chains but is sometimes discouraged by health specialists because of its high salt content. However, recent and ongoing research indicates that miso-containing diets may **lower** the risk of cardiovascular problems, despite the high salt content. Reasons for this are not yet totally clear but some researchers have speculated that the unique soy proteins that are formed when the beans are fermented is one of the key reasons. Also, miso is seldom eaten alone, so other cardio-protective foods (eg. rice, sea vegetables, onions, shitake mushrooms in soup) may play a role. Miso is also a rich source of tryptophan so a warming mug can be a quick and easy bedtime snack if you don't have time to make our *Turkey/Tofu & Spinach Soup.*

How Big is a Bowl?

Soup receptacles come in many different sizes and you have probably gleaned by now that we don't much like counting - and that includes portions. Little and often and eating until you are not quite full is the secret. When you eat regularly, get a good balance of essential nutrients in every snack and small meal and know that you are only a few hours away from your next plate or bowl of nourishment, it is a great deal easier to go small. If you are used to stuffing big portions down this can take a bit of practice but is an extremely worthwhile exercise so give it a go.

Brian Wansink, a Cornell University professor who spends much of his career doing brilliantly mischievous experiments based around the psychology of eating wrote a book, *Mindless Eating: Why We Eat More Than We Think* which I highly recommend. Over the years, he has done experiments with everything from different-sized plates and glasses to why we often lose track of how much we are eating when we are with friends and family but one experiment which is particularly pertinent here is his *Bottomless Soup Bowl* study. Participants were seated at a table, four at a time to eat soup but what they didn't know was that two of the four bowls were attached to a tube underneath the table which slowly and imperceptibly refilled the bowls. Those eating from the 'bottomless' bowls consumed an incredible 73 percent more soup than those eating from the normal bowls **and** estimated that they had consumed 140.5kcals fewer than they actually did. Those with the normal bowls reckoned they consumed only 32.3kcals fewer. And astonishingly, the 'bottomless' group didn't feel any fuller than the others! He believes, and many of his experiments clearly show that we often eat with our eyes and not with our stomachs and he offers a wealth of clever tips and tricks on how we can redress the balance. It's fascinating stuff and I would like to suggest that once you have read his book, the size of your soup receptacles and your portions will shrink along with your fat cells!

SOUP
RECIPES &
MORE

Ingredients in our Soups

A few guidelines on what we use in our soups:

- **Oils:** light olive oil, rapeseed oil, avocado oil and in Thai-Style soups, coconut oil for sautéing vegetables and browning meats. These are all less prone to damage when heated than oils that are high in polyunsaturated fats (sunflower, safflower, 'cooking' etc.)

- **Salt:** *Solo* low sodium salt or sea salt and celery salt for certain soups.

- **Pepper:** always freshly ground black pepper and occasionally white pepper for delicate soups.

- **Yoghurt:** 0% fat Greek or low fat natural yoghurts.

- **Stock:** we use our own when we have made a batch (see below) but we also regularly use good quality gels, pastes, cubes and cartons of fresh stock from the supermarket when time is tight which usually means we don't add salt to the soups.

- **Herbs:** mostly fresh and occasionally dried.

- **Garlic:** we love it and use it liberally and generally-speaking it doesn't leave traces of 'garlic breath' when cooked in soups but if you are not a garlic-lover or feel it is a little too much to handle early in the day, leave it out!

Protein Extras

As discussed in *Protein Packs a Punch* we recommend having a little protein with every meal and snack so all our soups that are predominantly vegetable-based include 'add a *Protein Extra*' at the end of the method. It's totally up to you whether you want to top your soup with a little protein or have a protein-rich snack on the side. Here are a few suggestions:

- Toasted nuts
- Toasted seeds
- Nut and Seed oils drizzled over before serving

- A decent dollop of 0% fat Greek yoghurt or low fat crème fraîche
- A dollop of hummus
- A good splash of anchovy essence or Gentleman's Relish
- Finely chopped cold boiled egg
- Cold cooked meats, poultry, game, fish or shellfish, finely sliced or diced

Talking Stock

Chicken or Meat Stock

Ingredients

4 chicken wings **or** ½ kg meat bones, roughly chopped
3 large sprigs parsley
1 leek, well-washed and roughly chopped
1 large onion, peeled and roughly chopped
2 carrots, peeled and roughly chopped
2 stalks celery, roughly sliced
½ teaspoon salt
½ teaspoon black peppercorns
2 bay leaves
1¼ litres water

Method

- Put all the ingredients into a large soup pot and bring slowly to the boil.
- Reduce the heat and simmer very gently for at least 2 hours (more if time allows).
- Pour through a fine sieve and allow the liquor to cool.
- Cover and place in the fridge overnight. This ensures that any fat solidifies on top and is quick and easy to remove with a slotted spoon.
- Keep what you are likely to use over the next 2-3 days in the fridge and freeze the rest in smaller portions or ice cube trays.
- When frozen, bag for future use.

Slow Cooker Chicken/Meat Stock

Put all the ingredients in the pot, stir well and cook on **low** for 8 hours. Strain and refrigerate/freeze as above.

Very Quick Chicken Stock

Ingredients

1 tablespoon oil
1 medium onion, peeled and roughly chopped
4 skinless chicken thighs
1 litre boiling water
1 teaspoon salt
1 bay leaf
1 bouquet garni

Method

* Warm the oil in a large soup pot.

* Add the onions and sauté gently until they are golden - don't let them burn.

* Remove the onions to a bowl.

* Turn up the heat and brown the chicken pieces on all sides.

* Return the onions to the pot, reduce the heat to low, cover and cook gently for 10-15 minutes until the chicken pieces release some of their juices.

* Increase the heat briefly whilst you add the boiling water, salt, bay leaf and bouquet garni then return to a very gentle simmer for about 25 minutes until the stock is rich and flavourful.

* Strain and use immediately or refrigerate overnight before reheating thoroughly and/or freeze in small containers or ice cube trays and once frozen, bag for future use.

Vegetable Stock

Ingredients

2 carrots, peeled and roughly chopped
1 red onion, peeled and roughly chopped
1 fennel bulb, trimmed and roughly chopped
3 celery stalks, roughly chopped
6 sprigs parsley
6 sprigs thyme
3cm piece fresh ginger, peeled and roughly chopped
4 cloves garlic, peeled and chopped
15 coriander seeds
10 black peppercorns
1 bay leaf
1 teaspoon salt
2 litres water

Method

- Put all the ingredients in a large soup pot.
- Bring slowly to the boil, reduce the heat and simmer very gently until all the vegetables are soft (35-45 minutes).
- Pass through a fine sieve. Don't mash the vegetables if you want a nice clear stock.
- For a richer broth, return the stock to the pot and cook briskly for a further 10-15 minutes to reduce.
- Let the stock cool to room temperature before refrigerating what you may use within 3 days or freeze in smaller portions or in ice cube trays.
- Once the cubes/portions are frozen, bag for future use.

Slow Cooker Vegetable Stock

Roasting the vegetables first makes a tasty stock.

Ingredients

6 carrots, scrubbed and roughly chopped
6 onions, peeled and roughly chopped
6 sticks celery, roughly chopped
450g mushrooms, cleaned and halved
6 cloves garlic, peeled and left whole
4 teaspoons oil
2.5 litres water
12 fresh parsley sprigs
15 black peppercorns
3 bay leaves
1 teaspoon salt

Method

- Preheat oven to 180C/350F/Gas Mark 4.
- Coat carrots, onions, celery, mushrooms and garlic in the oil and transfer to two shallow roasting tins.
- Roast until the vegetables are softened and browned but not burnt (about 40 minutes).
- Transfer to the slow cooker.
- Pour 250ml of the water into each roasting tin, heat, stirring and scraping up the browned bits from the tins then pour into the slow cooker.
- Add parsley, peppercorns, bay leaves, salt and the rest of the water to the slow cooker, cover and cook on **low** for 8 hours.
- Strain and refrigerate or freeze.

Very Quick Fish Stock

We don't come across many people who like messing around with fish heads, bones and skin but good fishmongers often make their own fish stock and sell it fresh so that is what we often opt for. We also use this simple, cheats method.

Ingredients

500g fresh or frozen white fish fillets (go for the cheapest)
1 leek, well washed and roughly chopped
1 carrot, scrubbed and roughly chopped
½ fennel bulb, trimmed and roughly chopped
1 garlic clove, peeled and chopped
3cm piece fresh ginger, peeled and chopped
A few sprigs of fresh tarragon, chervil or parley
6 black or mixed peppercorns
A couple of strips of lemon rind
3 tablespoons white wine (optional)
Salt

Method

- Defrost the fish fillets if using frozen.

- Put all the ingredients other than the salt in a large soup pot, cover with cold water and very slowly bring to just boiling.

- Reduce the heat to its lowest setting and simmer, covered for 20 minutes.

- Let the stock cool to room temperature then strain through a fine sieve.

- Season to taste and use immediately **or** refrigerate but use within one day **or** freeze in smaller portions or ice cube trays.

- Once frozen, bag the portions/cubes for future use.

- If using a slow cooker, cook on **low** for 4-6 hours.

Ready Made Stocks

All are likely to be higher in salt and salt equivalents than homemade stocks but as discussed, if you are including soup regularly in your diet, generally body swerving processed foods, buying and cooking fresh as often as possible and adding herbs, spices and natural flavourings along the way and heeding the advice outlined in *What's the Scoop on Salt?*, your daily salt consumption is likely to be within safe limits.

Generally speaking, fresh stocks in cartons/bags have the least amount of salt and added extras but they are reasonably pricey and don't have a very long shelf life. Cubes, pastes and gels are convenient and our advice is to opt for the more expensive varieties where possible and stay away from those which are super-cheap as they invariably involve rather a lot of health-disrupting MSG. Vegetable bouillon powders are also a good choice as they are often enriched with herbs and spices thus reducing the salt content.

SuperSkinny Soups

Gazpacho-Style Soup (without starch)

A fragrant and refreshingly light tomato soup/stew which is particularly good when warm rather than hot.

serves 2-3

Ingredients

6 medium, ripe tomatoes **or** 6 tinned tomatoes
1 large fennel bulb, trimmed, central stem removed then thinly sliced
450ml water
1 teaspoon salt
1 teaspoon coriander seeds
½ teaspoon black peppercorns
1 tablespoon oil
1 small onion, peeled and finely chopped
1 large clove garlic, peeled and crushed
½ tablespoon balsamic vinegar
1 tablespoon fresh lemon juice
2 heaped teaspoons fresh oregano leaves, finely chopped
1 heaped teaspoon tomato purée
Celery salt

Method

- Put the tomatoes in a large bowl, cover with boiling water, leave for 30 seconds then drain, remove the skins, stems and seeds and chop the flesh roughly.

- If you are using tinned tomatoes, remove the stems and seeds and chop the flesh roughly.

- Put the fennel and water in a small pot with the salt, bring slowly to the boil, reduce the heat, put a lid on and simmer very gently for 10-15 minutes or until the fennel is tender but still has a bite to it.

- Remove from the heat and set aside.

- Crush the coriander seeds and peppercorns in a pestle and mortar (ready-ground coriander and black pepper also work fine).

- Warm the oil in a large soup pot, add the onion and spices and sauté gently until the onions are soft (don't let them brown).

- Add the garlic and sauté for a further 5 minutes.

- Add the balsamic vinegar, lemon juice, chopped tomatoes, oregano and tomato puree and stir well.

- Add the fennel plus its simmering water, bring the soup to the boil then reduce the heat and simmer gently for 30 minutes.

- Remove from the heat and let it cool to room temperature before serving with a good shake of celery salt and a few chopped oregano leaves scattered over.

- Add a *Protein Extra*.

Very Quick Tomato Soup (without starch)

A soup, a drink, a **must** when you are in a rush.

serves 2

Ingredients

3 large ripe tomatoes **or** 3 tinned plum tomatoes
500ml fresh tomato juice
2 teaspoons Worcestershire sauce
2 teaspoons balsamic vinegar
Juice of 1 lime or half a lemon
4 drops Tabasco sauce
½ teaspoon celery salt
Pepper
0% fat Greek yoghurt
Mustard cress

Method

- If using fresh tomatoes, place them in a bowl, pour boiling water over and leave for 30 seconds.
- Drain, remove the skins, stalks and seeds and finely dice the flesh.
- If using tinned tomatoes, remove the stalks and seeds and finely chop the flesh.
- Put the tomato flesh, tomato juice, Worcester sauce, balsamic vinegar, lime/lemon juice, tabasco, celery salt and a few good grindings of pepper in a medium sized pot.
- Stir well and heat through until just beginning to boil.
- Taste and adjust, adding more of any of the flavourings and/or seasonings until it's just how you want it - some like it hot!
- Pour into bowls or mugs, top with a couple of good dollops of yoghurt per serving and scatter with snipped mustard cress or flask it if you are on the go.
- Adding a generous measure of Vodka on a lazy Saturday/Sunday morning can get the day off to a very cheering start!

Light Chicken Soup (with starch)

Fat busting, full of flavour and definitely 'good for the soul'.

serves 4

Ingredients

2 chicken thighs or 4 chicken wings
1 tablespoon oil
3 stalks celery, finely sliced
1 large onion, peeled and finely sliced
1 medium carrot, scrubbed and finely diced
1.2 litres chicken stock
100g brown rice
1 teaspoon horseradish sauce
3 stalks curly parsley, stalks removed and leaves finely chopped
Salt and pepper

Method

- Roast the chicken pieces in a medium to hot oven until the skins are crisp and the flesh is cooked through while you make the soup.

- If you made your own stock and have chicken pieces already cooked, shred/chop the flesh and put aside.

- Warm the oil, add the celery, onion and carrot and sauté gently until the vegetables are tender (about 15 minutes).

- Add the stock and bring slowly to the boil.

- Reduce the heat, add the rice and simmer, covered until the rice is cooked (around 30 minutes).

- Remove the chicken pieces to a board, skin and shred or chop the meat.

- Add the chicken, horseradish and parsley to the soup, stir well, heat through and season to taste before serving.

Chinese Little Gem & Chicken/Tofu Soup

(without starch)

A tasty, light broth with a warming kick.

serves 4

Ingredients

1 tablespoon oil
6-8 spring onions, white part very finely sliced, green part sliced into 1cm pieces
2 cloves garlic, peeled and very finely sliced or grated
2cm piece fresh ginger, peeled and very thinly sliced or grated
1 litre chicken or vegetable stock
2 skinless chicken breasts finely sliced along the grain or 300g smoked or unsmoked tofu, cubed (or use both - 1 chicken breast and 150g tofu)
A small red pepper, deseeded and very finely diced
2 little gem lettuce, shredded
1 teaspoon Tamari or light soy sauce
Salt and pepper

Method

- Warm the oil in a soup pot, add the white part of the spring onion, the garlic and the ginger and sauté gently for 10 minutes or until the onions are soft (don't let them brown).

- Add three quarters of the stock, bring slowly to the boil, reduce the heat then add the chicken and/or tofu, red pepper, the green part of the spring onion, lettuce and Tamari/soy sauce.

- Stir well and simmer gently for 8-10 minutes.

- Add the remainder of the stock if you like it more 'liquid', taste and season with salt and pepper if required before serving.

Spinach & Watercress Soup (with starch)

Lusciously green and because of the addition of oats, surprisingly filling.

serves 4

Ingredients

2 tablespoons oil
1 medium onion, peeled and finely chopped
800ml chicken or vegetable stock
1 heaped tablespoon porridge oats
2 bags spinach leaves
2 bags watercress
1 tablespoon fresh lemon juice
Salt and pepper

Method

- Warm the oil in a large soup pot and sauté the onion gently until soft.
- Add most of the stock and the porridge oats, bring slowly to the boil, reduce the heat and simmer for 15 minutes.
- Keep a good handful of the spinach leaves aside and add the remainder to the pot with the watercress.
- Keep stirring whilst bringing the soup back to the boil then turn off the heat.
- Liquidise the whole lot until you have a smooth, foamy soup then return to a clean pot.
- If it is a little too thick, add some or all of the remaining stock.
- Return to a clean pot, heat through gently, add the lemon juice and season to taste.
- Shred the spinach leaves you put aside and scatter over each bowl before serving.
- You can also grate a little lemon zest on top for added zing.
- Add a *Protein Extra*.

Beef Broth with Pearl Barley (with starch)

This has been a favourite with our fat busters for so long now it needs no explanation!

serves 4

Ingredients

1 tablespoon oil
300g lean stewing/chuck steak, cut into bite-sized chunks
1 tablespoon balsamic vinegar
1 tablespoon Worcestershire sauce
1 medium onion, peeled and finely chopped
3 carrots, peeled and diced
3 stalks celery, finely sliced
1 bay leaf
1 sprig fresh rosemary
2 litres beef stock
100g pearl barley, rinsed
Large handful fresh parsley leaves, roughly chopped
Salt and pepper

Method

- Warm the oil in a soup pot and quickly brown the meat over a high heat, stirring constantly.

- Add the balsamic vinegar and Worcestershire sauce and keep stirring until most of the liquid has evaporated.

- Reduce the heat and add the onion, carrots, celery, bay leaf and rosemary. Put the lid on and allow to gently sauté until the vegetables are tender.

- Add three quarters of the stock, bring to the boil, add the barley and parsley, stir well then reduce the heat and simmer for an hour or so until the barley and carrots are tender.

- Turn off the heat, remove the bay leaf and rosemary then whizz with a hand blender to slightly thicken but still leave a good chunky texture.

- Season to taste and if it is too thick add the remainder of the stock.

- This is one of those soups that thickens if left overnight as the barley continues to swell so check the consistency and add water if necessary before serving.

Pea Mint & Lettuce Soup (without starch)

Very quick, very colourful, very moreish, in no way seems like a 'slimming soup' and children love it!

serves 3

Ingredients

600ml frozen peas
600ml chicken or vegetable stock
1 old-fashioned round lettuce, cleaned and shredded
A generous bunch of fresh mint, chopped
Pepper
Natural yoghurt

Method

- Put a couple of handfuls of the peas in a bowl, pour over some boiling water and leave to plump up while you make the soup.
- Put the stock in a soup pot and bring to the boil.
- Add the remainder of the peas and simmer gently until tender.
- Turn off the heat and stir in the lettuce and mint.
- Whizz with a hand blender until smooth (or the texture you prefer) then return to a clean pot and reheat gently.
- Add a few good grindings of pepper (you are unlikely to need salt but taste and check).
- Ladle into bowls/mugs, top with a couple of teaspoons of yoghurt and quickly swirl with a skewer, drain the peas which have been soaking in the boiling water and scatter over the soup before serving.

Thai Curry Sweet Potato Soup (with starch)

Make it as spicy as you like and play around with the protein content to suit your tastes.

serves 4

Ingredients

250g sweet potato, peeled and chopped into dice-sized chunks
1 long thin red pepper, de-seeded and cut into fine strips
400ml tinned coconut milk
400ml chicken or vegetable stock
5 teaspoons thai red curry paste
12 fresh prawns **or** 1 skinless chicken breast cut into thin strips **or** chunks of tofu
Salt and pepper
50g fresh basil leaves, roughly chopped (also works well with baby spinach leaves)

Method

- Put the sweet potato, red pepper, coconut milk, stock and curry paste into a large soup pot, stir well and bring slowly to the boil.

- Reduce the heat and simmer for 20 minutes or until the sweet potato is tender and just beginning to fall apart - this will thicken the soup. You can thicken the soup further by mashing the sweet potato slightly if you wish.

- Add your protein of choice and stir over a low heat to cook through. The prawns and tofu will only take a couple of minutes, the chicken slightly longer.

- Season to taste.

- Stir in the basil leaves and when just wilted, serve the soup.

- You can add more curry paste before adding the protein if you like a bit more spice.

Spicy Meatball Soup (without starch)

Quite a lot of ingredients here but very well-worth the little extra time and effort.

serves 4

Ingredients

400g lean minced beef, lamb or chicken
1 egg, lightly whisked
2 tablespoons fresh herbs, finely chopped (parsley/oregano/thyme/marjoram)
½ teaspoon salt
a few good grindings of black pepper
Pinch chilli powder
1 tablespoon oil
1 large onion, peeled and finely chopped
2 large carrots, peeled and finely diced
1 large stalk celery, finely sliced
1 small red chilli, deseeded and finely diced
1 large clove garlic, peeled and crushed
1 large courgette, sliced or chopped
1 heaped tablespoon tomato puree
1 litre beef/chicken/lamb stock (depending on your choice of meat)
1 x 400g tinned, chopped tomatoes
100g curly kale/savoy cabbage, very finely sliced
Salt and pepper
Good bunch fresh parsley, chopped

Method

- Thoroughly mix the minced meat/poultry, egg, herbs, salt, pepper and chilli powder in a bowl with a fork.

- Make around 16 bite-sized meatballs with your hands, lay them on a dish, cover and put in the fridge while you make the soup.

- Heat the oil in a large soup pot, add the onion, carrot and celery and sauté gently until the onion is soft and translucent and the carrots are slightly tender (don't brown).

- Add the chilli, garlic, courgette and tomato puree, stir well and sauté for a further 5 minutes.
- Add the stock and tinned tomatoes, bring slowly to the boil, reduce the heat and simmer for 15 minutes or until the carrots are tender.
- Add the kale/cabbage and simmer for a further 5 minutes.
- Add the meatballs to the soup with a large spoon and simmer gently until they are cooked through (around 8-10 minutes).
- Check the seasoning and serve; 4 meatballs to a bowl, topped with lots of fresh parsley.

Turkey/Tofu & Spinach Soup (with starch)

Nothing like it for a restful and restorative night's sleep.

serves 4

Ingredients

1 turkey drumstick, skin removed
1 litre chicken stock
85g white basmati rice, rinsed
100g spinach leaves, washed and roughly chopped
Salt and pepper

Method

- Place the turkey leg in a large soup pot, add the stock and slowly bring to the boil.
- Reduce the heat and simmer for 30-40 minutes, covered until the turkey meat is cooked through.
- Add the rice and simmer for a further 15 minutes or until the rice is cooked and soft.
- Remove the turkey leg, pull the meat from the bone then shred with a couple of forks or chop into bite-sized chunks.
- Add the spinach and turkey meat to the broth and simmer for a few more minutes until the spinach has wilted but the leaves are still silky.
- Season to taste and serve.

Vegetarian Alternative

Ingredients

1 litre vegetable stock
85g white basmati rice, rinsed
300g tofu, cubed
100g spinach leaves, washed and roughly chopped

Method

- Place the stock in a large soup pot and slowly bring to the boil.
- Add the rice and simmer for 15 minutes or until the rice is cooked and soft.
- Add the tofu and simmer for a further 10 minutes.
- Toss in the spinach and stir until the leaves have wilted but are still silky.
- Season to taste and serve.

Instant and Ready-Made Soups

Miso Soup: Sachets or pastes with boiling water added or ready-made.

Vegetable Bouillon Powders: Dissolve in a mug of boiling water and add a *Protein Extra*.

Light Broths and Consommes: Chicken, turkey, beef, vegetable.

Green Soups: Spinach, watercress, lettuce, courgettes etc. Stay away from those with cream and add a *Protein Extra*.

Skinny Soups

Spicy Turkey Soup (without starch)

If you like a little less spice, leave out the chilli - a great meal in a bowl.

serves 4

Ingredients

1 tablespoon oil
1 large clove garlic, peeled and crushed
1 red chilli, deseeded and finely chopped
1 onion, peeled and finely chopped
1 bunch (6-8) spring onions, finely sliced
Small pack of pancetta cubes or 75g lean bacon, diced
½ tsp dried oregano
Pinch cayenne pepper
Pinch ground cumin
1 x 400g tin peeled chopped tomatoes
1 litre chicken or vegetable stock
1 bay leaf
1 small turkey drumstick or 2 chicken drumsticks, skin off
3 tablespoons frozen peas and corn
Salt and pepper
1 good handful fresh coriander or parsley leaves, chopped
Fresh lime juice

Method

- Warm the oil in a soup pot, add the garlic, chilli, onion and spring onions and sauté gently for 10-15 minutes until the onions are soft and translucent (don't let them brown).

- In a small frying pan, sauté the pancetta/bacon until it is just browned around the edges and drain on kitchen paper before adding to the soup pot.

- Add the oregano, cayenne pepper and cumin and stir well.

- Add the tomatoes, stock, bay leaf, turkey/chicken drumsticks and bring slowly to the boil.

- Reduce the heat and simmer gently until the meat is cooked and falling off the bone (around 35 minutes).
- Add the peas and corn and simmer for a further 8-10 minutes.
- Remove the bay leaf, transfer the drumstick/s to a board and shred the cooked meat with a couple of forks before returning to the pot for a couple of minutes to warm through.
- Season to taste, top each bowl of soup with the coriander/parsley and add a splash of fresh lime juice before serving.

Thai Prawn Noodle Soup (with or without starch)

Absolutely delicious and a gorgeous colour. Very quickly becomes a staple!

serves 4 to 5

Ingredients

2 red chillies, deseeded and roughly chopped
6 shallots, peeled and roughly chopped
3 cloves garlic, peeled
5cm piece of fresh ginger, peeled and roughly chopped
1 stalk lemon grass, bashed and sliced
1 teaspoon ground turmeric
1 teaspoon ground coriander
10g fresh parsley or coriander leaves
2 tablespoons oil
2 x 400ml tins coconut milk
400ml fish stock
2 tablespoons fish sauce (nam plah)
2 x 220g bags of frozen raw king prawns
150g thin cooked rice noodles (optional)
Salt and pepper
Juice of half a lime

Method

- Blitz the chillies, shallots, garlic, ginger, lemongrass, turmeric, ground coriander, fresh parsley/coriander and oil in a food processor and whizz until you have a smooth paste.

- Transfer to a soup pot and cook over a very gentle heat for 5 minutes.

- Add the coconut milk and stock, bring to the boil, reduce the heat and simmer gently for 10 minutes.

- Add the fish sauce and prawns and simmer, stirring for a further 5 minutes.

- Add the noodles, if using and slowly bring back to the boil.

- Turn off the heat, season to taste, add the lime juice and let the soup stand for a couple of minutes before serving.

Adzuki Bean Soup (with starch)

Sling it all into the slow cooker if you have one and hey presto! Quick, easy and satisfying even if you don't.

serves 4

Ingredients

1 x 400g tin Adzuki beans
1 x 400g tin chopped tomatoes
450mls chicken/vegetable stock
1 onion, peeled and finely chopped
2 garlic cloves, peeled and crushed
1 red pepper, deseeded and finely chopped
8 button mushrooms, roughly sliced or chopped
1 tablespoon tomato puree
1 teaspoon smoked or unsmoked paprika powder
A very generous splash of Worcestershire Sauce
Salt and pepper
2 tablespoons fresh parsley leaves, roughly chopped

Method

- Put all the ingredients other than the salt, pepper and parsley into your slow cooker, stir well and cook on **low** for about 5 hours.

- Season to taste and add more paprika and/or Worcestershire Sauce and salt and pepper if required before serving topped with the parsley.

- If you don't have a slow cooker, gently sauté the onion, garlic and red pepper in a tablespoon of oil in a large soup pot until soft. Add the remainder of the ingredients other than the salt, pepper and parsley, bring slowly to the boil, reduce the heat and simmer very gently for 30 minutes.

- Season to taste and add more paprika and/or Worcestershire Sauce and salt and pepper if required before serving topped with the parsley.

- Add a *Protein Extra*.

Tomato Soup (without starch)

Looks remarkably like tinned tomato soup but is way more delicious and there's no sugar!

serves 4

Ingredients

1 tablespoon oil
1 medium onion, peeled and finely chopped
1 stalk celery, finely chopped
2 x 400g tins chopped tomatoes
6cm strip of lemon rind
1 bouquet garni
1 litre chicken or vegetable stock
150ml dry sherry (optional)
Salt and pepper
Celery leaves or fresh parsley leaves, finely chopped

Method

- Warm the oil in a soup pot and gently sauté the onion and celery until soft.
- Add the tomatoes, lemon rind, bouquet garni and stock and bring slowly to the boil.
- Reduce the heat and simmer for 25 minutes.
- Add the sherry is using and simmer for a further 10 minutes.
- Remove the lemon rind and bouquet garni, transfer to a liquidiser and blitz until the soup is very smooth (to make it even smoother, pass the soup through a sieve before returning to the pot).
- Reheat, season to taste and serve topped with the celery or parsley leaves.
- If you prefer a chunkier texture, remove the lemon rind and bouquet garni then just roughly blitz the soup in the pot with a hand blender.
- Add a *Protein Extra*.

Carrot & Saffron Soup with Tomato Crisps

(without starch)

Delicate and delicious and great for entertaining. A beautiful soup with a sweet and sour edge. Thanks to Mo Scott who introduced us to this soup. A great cook and an inspiration to all.

serves 4-6

Ingredients

6 small ripe tomatoes
12-15 saffron threads
2 tablespoons oil
450g carrots, peeled and diced
1 large onion, peeled and finely chopped
1 clove garlic, peeled and finely chopped
1 level teaspoon ground cumin
2 level teaspoons ground coriander
1 litre chicken or vegetable stock
Salt and pepper
Juice of half an orange
1 level teaspoon whole cumin seeds
Low fat crème fraîche

Method

- Make the tomato crisps the day/night before if using (not essential, but a pretty addition and intensely tasty). See below for method.

- Put the saffron threads in 2 tablespoons warm water and leave aside.

- Warm the oil in a soup pot, add the carrots, onion and garlic and sauté gently until they begin to soften (don't brown).

- Add the cumin and coriander and stir for a few minutes until very fragrant.

- Add the strained saffron liquor and the stock and bring slowly to the boil.

- Reduce the heat and simmer, uncovered for 30 minutes or until the carrots are very tender.

- Transfer to a liquidiser and blitz until the soup is very smooth and frothy. Pass through a sieve if you have time before returning to a clean pot.

- Heat through, season to taste and add the orange juice.
- To serve, dry-fry the cumin seeds briefly in a small frying pan until they begin to pop.
- Ladle the soup into bowls, top each with a good dollop of crème fraîche and scatter with a few roasted cumin seeds and the tomato crisps.

Tomato Crisps

- Heat the oven to its lowest setting.
- Thinly slice the tomatoes, discarding the end slices and place the rest on kitchen foil brushed with a little olive oil on a roasting tray. Don't let the slices touch.
- Place in the middle of the oven and leave until the tomatoes are crisp and dry (around 5-7 hours). Test one by snapping it in half.
- The colour will have dulled slightly but the slices will be glossy. Lift them off the foil carefully with a spatula.

Lamb & Bean Soup (with starch)

This is a soup that warms you from top to toe, delivers a bucketload of nourishment and works really well when flasked and taken on-the-road. Fiona's husband's favourite - one bowl is simply never enough!

serves 4

Ingredients

4 medium, ripe tomatoes **or** 4 tinned plum tomatoes
1 x 400g tin black-eyed or canellini beans
250g lean minced lamb
1 tablespoon Worcestershire sauce
1 teaspoon ground cumin
1 teaspoon paprika powder
1 teaspoon chilli powder
1 tablespoon oil
1 large onion, peeled and finely chopped
2 carrots, scrubbed and cut into thin strips
1 long red pepper, deseeded and cut into thin strips
2 cloves garlic, peeled and finely chopped
400ml lamb or vegetable stock
¼ Savoy cabbage, finely sliced
Salt and pepper
Parsley or coriander leaves, chopped finely

Method

- Put the tomatoes in a bowl, pour boiling water over, leave for 30 seconds then drain, skin, remove the stalks, deseed and chop the flesh roughly. Put aside.
- If you are using tinned tomatoes, remove the stalks and seeds and roughly chop the flesh.
- Drain the beans, reserving the liquid, put two-thirds of the beans aside and liquidise the remaining third with their liquid until smooth.
- Very quickly brown the meat over a fairly high heat in a non-stick pan.
- Add the Worcestershire sauce and keep stirring until the meat absorbs the liquid.

- Add the spices and stir well for a couple more minutes before removing the pan from the heat.
- Warm the oil in a large soup pot, add the onion and carrot and sauté until tender.
- Add the red pepper and garlic and sauté for a further 5 minutes.
- Add the liquidised beans, stock and lamb mince to the pot, bring slowly to the boil then reduce the heat and simmer gently for 10 minutes.
- Add the tomato flesh (keep a few teaspoons back for topping the soup before serving if you wish), the remaining beans and the cabbage and simmer for a further 10 minutes or until the cabbage is tender but still has a bite to it.
- Check the seasoning before serving topped with parsley/coriander.

Smoked Haddock & White Bean Soup
(with starch)

Very quick, very creamy, very tasty and even non-fish lovers have been known to dig in with enthusiasm!

serves 4

Ingredients

4-6 saffron strands
1 tablespoon oil
2 large onions, peeled and finely chopped
1 x 400g tin haricot/cannellini beans, drained and rinsed
750ml fish or vegetable stock
250g smoked haddock fillet, skinned and cut into bite-sized pieces
A handful of finely chopped fresh parsley leaves or chopped chives

Method

*   Put the saffron strands in a cup, pour over a little warm water and leave aside.
*   Warm the oil in a large soup pot, add the onions and sauté gently until soft - don't let them brown or the soup won't end up a lovely, creamy colour.
*   Add the beans and stock, bring slowly to the boil, reduce the heat and simmer for 15 minutes.
*   Strain the saffron, add the liquor to the pot and stir well.
*   Add the smoked haddock and continue to simmer for a further 5 minutes or until the fish is cooked and flakes easily.
*   Either liquidise the whole lot until very smooth **or** remove the pieces of fish and liquidise the rest before returning both to a clean pan **or** give the soup 4 to 5 good circular blasts with a hand blender to produce a chunky texture.
*   Top with the parsley/chives before serving.

Mushroom Soup (without starch)

Intensely mushroomy and can be served in a number of different ways.

serves 4

Ingredients

20g dried porcini mushrooms
1 tablespoon oil
2 medium onions, peeled and finely sliced or chopped
600g button mushrooms, cleaned and finely sliced or chopped
1 litre chicken or vegetable stock
1 tablespoon Mushroom Ketchup
100ml dry sherry (optional)
Salt and pepper
Fresh parsley leaves, chopped

Method

- Soak the dried mushrooms in 200ml boiling water and set aside while you get on with preparing the onions and button mushrooms.
- Warm the oil in a large soup pot, add the onion and sauté for 10 minutes until golden.
- Add the fresh mushrooms and sauté for a further 5 minutes.
- Drain the dried mushrooms, keeping the soaking liquor, roughly chop the mushrooms and add both to the pot.
- Add the stock, Mushroom Ketchup and sherry, if using and gently simmer for 15 minutes.
- Season to taste.
- At this stage you can either serve the soup as it is, liquidise the whole lot until smooth and creamy **or** remove the mushrooms before liquidising the rest then return both to a clean pot before reheating and serving with loads of parsley.
- Add a *Protein Extra*.

Crab & Ginger Soup (without starch)

Velvety smooth, deliciously fishy and great for entertaining.

serves 4

Ingredients

2 tablespoons oil
1 medium onion, peeled and finely chopped
2 cloves garlic, peeled and finely chopped
5cm piece fresh ginger, peeled and finely chopped
2 tablespoons brandy (optional)
2 tablespoons tomato puree
750ml fish stock
140g fresh white fish fillets, roughly chopped
225g fresh white crab meat (good quality tinned crab also works fine)
Salt and pepper
Fresh dill

Method

- Warm the oil in a soup pot over a low heat, add the onion, garlic and ginger and gently sauté with the lid on for 10 minutes.

- Add the brandy if using, turn up the heat a little and reduce until most of the liquid has gone (this burns off the alcohol).

- Add the tomato puree and stir well before adding the stock then bring slowly to the boil.

- Reduce the heat, add the white fish, stir well and simmer very gently for 10 minutes.

- Add the crab meat and continue to simmer for a further 5 minutes.

- Liquidise until you have a very smooth soup, return to a clean pot and reheat slowly.

- Season to taste and serve, adding a few dill fronds to each bowl.

Beetroot Soup (without starch)

You may think you don't like beetroot but just try this soup and you will be won over!

serves 4

Ingredients

500g fresh beetroot, left whole, washed but not peeled
1 tablespoon oil
2 large carrots, peeled and diced
2 stalks celery, finely sliced
2 large red onions, peeled and finely chopped
750ml chicken or vegetable stock
4 stalks fresh parsley, stalks removed and leaves finely chopped
Juice of half a lemon
Salt and pepper
Crème fraîche (optional)

Method

- Put the beetroot in a large pot and cover with 1 litre of cold water.
- Bring to the boil then reduce the heat and simmer until tender (around 45 minutes).
- Turn off the heat and leave the beetroot to cool in the water.
- Warm the oil in a soup pot and gently sauté the carrots, celery and onion for 10 minutes or until softened.
- When the beetroot are cool, remove from the water, put on a pair of rubber gloves, slip off the skins, dice the flesh and add to the soup pot along with the stock and the parsley (keep some parsley aside for topping if you wish).
- Bring to the boil then reduce the heat and simmer gently for 30 minutes or until all the vegetables are tender.
- Add the lemon juice little by little and keep tasting until you are happy with the sharp/sweet flavour balance.
- You can leave the soup as it is or gently mash or blend to your desired texture.

- Season and serve. Top each bowl with a dollop of crème fraîche, if using and the remaining parsley if you kept some aside.

- Add a *Protein Extra* if you are not using the crème fraîche as a topping.

- For speed, the soup also works well with ready-cooked fresh beetroot (not the stuff in vinegar!)

FatBustForever Soups

Pea & Ham Soup (with starch)

A meal in a bowl but unlike many pea and ham soup recipes, it's surprisingly light. Warning! It's hard to restrict yourself to just one bowl!

serves 4

Ingredients

2 tablespoons oil
1 large onion, peeled and finely chopped
2 large carrots, scrubbed and finely diced
1 celery stick, finely sliced
Pepper
3 bay leaves
500g green split peas, rinsed
1 ham hock/pork knuckle
300g green cabbage, finely shredded

Method

- Heat the oil in a large soup pot, add the onion, carrot and celery and gently sauté for about 15 minutes until the vegetables are softened.

- Season well with pepper, add the bay leaves and peas and stir well.

- Add the ham hock, cover with cold water and bring slowly to the boil.

- Reduce the heat and simmer for 2 hours.

- When the meat is falling of the bone, take it out and after removing the fat, pick all the meat from the bone and chop finely or shred with a couple of forks.

- Remove the bay leaves from the soup then add the ham meat along with the cabbage.

- Continue to simmer until the cabbage is cooked, check the seasoning and serve.

- If you have time, let the soup cool and refrigerate overnight. Next day, remove the fat from the top and reheat.

- If you have a slow cooker, put all the ingredients in the pot and cook on **low** for 6-8 hours or **high** for 4-6 hours before removing the ham and following the method above.

- If the soup is too thick, add a little water.

Lamb Tagine Soup (with or without starch)

This fragrant and meaty soup transports you to Morocco in super quick time. You can leave out the rice for a still very tasty non starchy soup.

serves 4

Ingredients

1 tablespoon oil
250g lean lamb shoulder, cut into bite-sized chunks
½ tsp paprika
½ tsp ground ginger (or a good teaspoon of grated fresh ginger)
½ tsp ground cinnamon
½ tsp ground turmeric
1 leek, well-washed and finely sliced
2 medium-sized parsnips, peeled, woody stem removed and diced
2 large carrots, peeled and diced
½ cooking apple, peeled, cored and diced
1 litre lamb or vegetable stock
1 x 400g tin chopped tomatoes
30g brown rice
4 good sprigs of fresh parsley, stems removed and leaves roughly chopped
Salt and pepper

Method

- Warm the oil in a soup pot and quickly brown the lamb over a medium heat.
- Add the paprika, ginger, cinnamon and turmeric and stir well to coat the lamb.
- Add the leek, parsnip, carrot and apple, stir well then reduce the heat to low, put the lid on and allow everything to sauté gently for 10-15 minutes.
- Add most of the stock, the tomatoes and the rice, bring to the boil then reduce the heat and simmer for 40 minutes or until the rice is cooked and the carrots are very tender.
- Add the remainder of the stock if the soup is too thick.

- Add the parsley, stir for a couple of minutes, season to taste and serve as it is or use the hand blender to mash the soup a bit.

- If you are keeping the soup until the next day you may have to add more stock/water as the rice will have plumped up and thickened it.

Minestrone (with starch)

A minestrone is 'a thick soup with vegetables' so you can really play around with this soup and use whatever is in the cupboard, fridge or freezer. Here is ours!

serves 4

Ingredients

1 tablespoon oil
4 rashers very lean smoked bacon, chopped or a small packet of cubed pancetta
1 red onion, peeled and finely chopped
1 carrot, peeled and diced
1 stick celery, finely sliced
1 leek, well-washed and finely sliced
2 cloves garlic, peeled and finely sliced/chopped
1 x 400g tin chopped tomatoes
1 large courgette, diced
½ Savoy or green cabbage, finely shredded
750ml ham, chicken or vegetable stock
1 bouquet garni
1 x 400g tin red kidney beans, drained and well-rinsed
Small bunch fresh basil, roughly chopped
200g spinach leaves, roughly chopped
Salt and pepper

Method

- Warm the oil in a large soup pot and add the bacon/pancetta, onion, carrot, celery, leek and garlic.
- Sauté over a gentle heat until the vegetables are soft, around 15 minutes.
- Add the tomatoes, courgette, cabbage, stock and bouquet garni and bring slowly to the boil.
- Reduce the heat and simmer gently for 15 minutes or until the carrot is very tender.
- Add the kidney beans and simmer for a further 10 minutes then add the basil and spinach.

- When the basil and spinach have just wilted, remove the bouquet garni, season to taste and serve.
- Add more stock/water if the soup is too thick.
- If you prefer pasta in your minestrone, replace the red kidney beans with 50g small macaroni (add at the same time as the stock) or orzo (add at the point where you would add the beans).

Scotch Broth (with starch)

There's nothing like it on a cold day - it really sticks to your ribs and fills you up! A soup you never tire of.

serves 4

Ingredients

90g broth mix
1.7 litres beef stock
1 small shin/shank of beef **or** 250g stewing/chuck steak in a piece
1 tablespoon Worcestershire sauce
1 large leek, well-washed and finely sliced
1 stalk celery, finely sliced
2 large carrots, peeled and diced
1 x 400g tin cooked butter beans, drained and rinsed
1 large bunch fresh parsley, stems removed and leaves roughly chopped
Salt and pepper

Method

- Soak the broth mix in cold water overnight, drain and rinse.
- Put the stock in a soup pot and bring slowly to the boil, add the broth mix, beef, Worcestershire sauce, leek, celery and carrot and bring back to the boil.
- Reduce the heat to a very low setting and simmer for 1 hour or until the meat is very tender and the vegetables are cooked.
- Take the meat out, remove the fat and chop or shred with 2 forks.
- Add the butter beans, meat and parsley to the pot and bring the soup back to the boil.
- Reduce the heat and simmer for a further 10 minutes.
- Season to taste and serve.
- Like many broths, this soup is better on the second day. Add water whilst reheating if it is too thick.

Roasted Tomato, Red Pepper & Chorizo Soup
(with or without starch)

This soup won't disappoint. It is colourful, filling and intensely flavoured and you can use all kinds of different beans and spicy/smoked sausages to create your own special favourite.

serves 4

Ingredients

1 red onion, unpeeled and quartered
2 long sweet red peppers, de-seeded and halved lengthways
4 tomatoes
2 garlic cloves, unpeeled
500ml chicken stock
400g can red kidney/cannellini beans, drained and rinsed
100g chorizo or smoked sausage, cut into bite-sized chunks
2 teaspoons balsamic vinegar
Salt and pepper
15g fresh basil or parsley leaves, chopped

Method

- Preheat the oven to 180C/350F/Gas Mark 4.
- Put the onions, peppers, tomatoes and garlic in a large bowl, drizzle in a little oil and stir well before arranging the vegetables on a baking sheet, cut sides down.
- Roast for 15-20 minutes or until the onions are cooked through. Remove the skins from the onions and peppers and the skin and seeds from the tomatoes. Placing the peppers in a plastic bag for 5 minutes makes the peeling very quick and easy.
- Chop half the vegetables into small chunks and set aside.
- Put the rest of the vegetables into a food processor or blender with the garlic squeezed from its skin and the stock.
- Process until smooth then transfer to a soup pot with the chopped vegetables you put aside.
- Bring the soup slowly to the boil, stirring occasionally.
- Add the beans, chorizo or smoked sausage and balsamic vinegar,

reduce the heat, cover and simmer gently for 10 minutes.

- Season to taste.
- Toss in the basil/parsley and give the soup a good stir before serving.
- Also works well if you peel and chop all the vegetables and sauté in 1 tablespoon of oil until soft instead of roasting.
- You can leave out the red kidney beans for a non-starchy soup.

Mulligatawny (with starch)

A peppery soup with curry undertones which has a load of history behind it - this is our version.

serves 4

Ingredients

1 tablespoon oil
1 lamb shank or 1 turkey drumstick
1 large onion, peeled and finely chopped
1 large carrot, peeled and diced
1 large parsnip, peeled, woody centre removed and diced
50g brown basmati rice
2 tablespoons curry powder
1 litre lamb or chicken stock (depending on your choice of meat)
1 large Granny Smith apple, peeled, cored and diced
Salt and pepper

Method

- Heat the oil in a large soup pot and quickly brown the lamb/turkey on all sides over a medium heat.

- Add the onion and brown for 5 minutes then add the carrot and parsnip and brown for a further 5 minutes.

- Add the rice and curry powder and stir well until fragrant.

- Add most of the stock, bring to the boil then reduce the heat and simmer for 25 minutes.

- Add the apple and simmer for a further 20 minutes or until the vegetables are tender, the rice is cooked and the meat is falling off the bone.

- Take the meat out, remove the skin, pick off the meat and chop or shred with 2 forks before returning to the soup and warming through.

- Season to taste and if you have time, let the soup cool and refrigerate overnight. Next day, remove any fat from the top, reheat and serve.

- If time is tight you can use diced beef, lamb, turkey or chicken and reduce the simmering time. Just make sure the meat/poultry are very tender and beginning to fall apart and the rice is cooked before serving.

In a Rush, On the Go and Eating Out Soups

When you are in SuperSkinny Mode

Bit of vigilance is required here and remember to always add a *Protein Extra* if there is no protein in the soup.

- **Miso Soup:** Sachets or pastes with boiling water added or ready-made.
- **Vegetable Bouillon Powders:** Dissolve in a mug of boiling water.
- **Light Broths and Consommes:** Chicken, turkey, beef, vegetable.
- **Green Soups:** Spinach, watercress, lettuce, courgettes etc. Stay away from those with cream.

When you are in Skinny Mode and Beyond

- Aim for soups that have a nutrition label giving you the sugar, saturated fat and salt levels.
- If you have a favourite soup haunt or a favourite range of soups, look at the websites and check the nutritional status so you know which ones to choose.
- The fresher the soup the less processed it is so those with a short shelf life are often your best bet.
- Select those with a short list of **real and recognisable** food ingredients.
- Body swerve 'diet' soups, most of them are tasteless and ghastly and a quick look at the ingredients says it all!
- Be on your guard with tinned soups - too many preservatives, natural or otherwise and some of them have been on the shelves for months.

How to read the label. Look at the *per 100g* column rather than the *per serving* column and aim for:

- Carbohydrates, *of which sugars* - maximum 4g
- Fats, *of which saturates* - maximum 2g
- Salt or *salt equivalent* - maximum 0.6g
- Sodium - maximum 0.2g

Don't get hung up on the calorie column. If you stick to the above recommendations you will be getting the best possible quality calories from a ready-made soup. For fat loss you need nourishment not a calculator.

Best Choice Soups Off the Shelf for Continued Fat Loss

Again, check the labels where possible and only have the ones with top notch starchy carbohydrates before 6pm unless you exercise in the evening. Watch out for words like *Big*, *Hearty*, *Healthy*, *Stay Full*, *Skinny*, *Light*, *Slim*, *Trim* and *Low* on the pack. Most have added extras and a list of ingredients as long as your arm. Having said that, some small manufacturers of lovingly-prepared and delicious fresh soups seem to feel the need to add the odd weight loss promises on the label rather than just promoting them as great soups, which many of them are - that'll be the marketing men at work, no doubt!

If you are having a predominantly vegetable soup, have a *Protein Extra* topping or on the side.

- Miso Soups
- Vegetable Soups
- Meaty Soups (beef, lamb)
- Game Soups (venison, rabbit, pheasant)
- Chicken and Turkey Broths
- Broths with Meatballs
- Fish and Shellfish Soups (not chowders)
- Spicy Soups
- Curry Soups
- Thai Soups
- Moroccan Soups
- Squash Soups
- Bean Soups
- Lentil Soups

- Chickpea Soups
- Soups with a little rice or barley

There are always going to be soups where you simply don't know or can't find out the sugar, saturated fat and salt levels or how much starchy carbohydrate is involved but as long as you have them occasionally and not daily, you shouldn't get into too much trouble. Equally, some soups with labels may not fit within the above recommendations but as long as only **one** of the three S's is over the maximum and not all three and the soup is not mega-dense with rice, potato or pasta you can take a reasonably relaxed approach. The big secret is to go for variety and not stick to the same soups day after day.

Worst Choice Soups Off the Shelf for Continued Fat Loss

Avoid those that include the following in the title or the description:

- Pasta, noodles or starchy dumplings
- Cheese
- Corn/Sweetcorn
- Sausage
- Potato
- Croutons
- Cream of...
- Chowder
- Bisques
- Luxury

Non-Soup Breakfasts and Early Morning Choices

- **Eggs:** two boiled, poached or scrambled eggs on or with rye toast.
- **Bacon:** two rashers of lean bacon, two grilled tomatoes and two large grilled mushrooms.
- **Hummus:** two large oatcakes slathered with hummus and topped with sliced tomato.
- **Porridge:** a bowl of porridge made with water topped with a swirl of runny honey, sliced fresh apple and a good sprinkling of cinnamon.
- **Smoothies:** homemade if you have time using whatever is in the fruit bowl with a couple of spoonfuls of natural yoghurt and a tablespoon of flax seed oil added or bought if time is tight (go for the ones with added yoghurt or have a little pot of yoghurt alongside those that don't).
- **Toast and Butter:** two slices of rye bread, toasted and spread with nut or seed butter (almond, hazelnut, cashew, peanut, pumpkin seed, sunflower seed) and topped with fresh fruit slices or no sugar jam.
- **Ham, Cheese and Melon:** wrap a few slices of cooked or Parma ham around chunks of goats cheese cheddar and melon slices - very quick, very filling.

Non-Soup Super Quick Snacks

Keep some of the following in your handbag, briefcase, glove compartment, desk drawer, cupboard, fridge and fruit bowl and remember that **a small snack is all that is required to keep you nourished and satisfied until you next eat**. Aim to have one item from each list to get a good balance of carbohydrates, protein and fat:

- Oatcakes
- Ryvita/rye crackers
- Rice cakes

- Cooked cold meats
- Cooked chicken/turkey

- Smoked fish
- Tinned oily fish
- Fresh cooked prawns, shrimps, crab
- Hard cheese, goats cheese, cottage cheese
- Boiled hens eggs or quails eggs
- Hummus, tzatsiki, taramasalata, guacamole
- 0% fat Greek yoghurt
- Mixed bean salad
- Lentil salad

- Avocado
- Apples and pears
- Cherries and berries
- Bananas
- Chopped fruit selections
- Raw vegetable selections.
- Tomatoes.
- Baby gem lettuce
- Vegetables in oil (peppers, artichokes, aubergines, sun dried tomatoes)

- Nuts
- Seeds
- Nut and Seed butters

If you are horribly short of time and the selection isn't great have a bag of nuts and/or seeds and a piece of fruit or if all else fails, a cereal bar. The majority of them are marketed as *healthy snacks* but few fit the brief. There is sometimes more sugar than in a good-sized bar of creamy milk chocolate - label reading is a must here!

WEIGHTS

MEASURES &

INGREDIENTS

Another great thing about soups is that exact measurements are not vital (unlike baking!) We use litres and millilitres for fluids and grams, UK tablespoons and teaspoons for dry ingredients in all our recipes but are well aware that equivalents in other countries can cause a bit of recipe confusion. We also use UK food names so if you are used to cooking with eggplant, zucchini and cilantro you may wonder what aubergine, courgette and coriander are!

A lady by the name of Annie, a keen cook who came from the US to the UK some number of years ago and found it difficult to follow a British recipe has gone to enormous lengths to clarify cooking temperatures, weights and measures and food name equivalents and post them on a website.

We haven't been able to track her down but if you are reading this Annie, thank you for what must have been a long and arduous task!

Visit www.goo.gl/dtkci for cooking temperatures, weights and measures.
Visit www.goo.gl/zPYb8 for food name equivalents.

There are many other websites dedicated to providing similar information for other countries - seek them out.

It is also impossible to come up with recipes that include seasonal ingredients from every corner of the globe when some readers are basking in crazy hot temperatures while others are trudging through snow and ice. Equally, every country has its own unique cuisine and certain foods play a major role. Jean and I are Scottish and our soups often reflect our heritage and champion ingredients that we have learned to love since childhood but we both have a very global approach to food and are keen to learn more about soup ingredients, cooking methods and different ways of creating new and exciting soups. We are always on a soup journey and urge you, wherever you are to share your favourite recipes, tips and general soup chat on our website, www.souperydupery.com.

Books by Fiona Kirk

www.fatbustforever.com

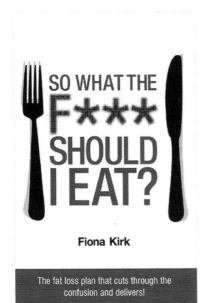

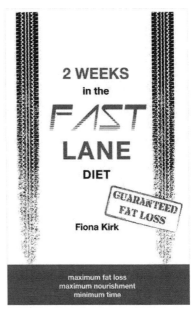

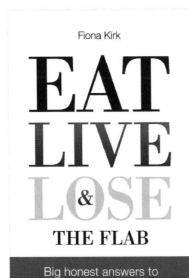

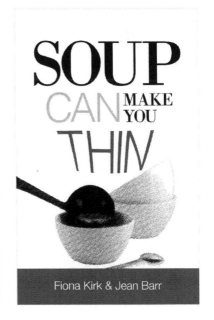

References

- Rolls BJ, Bell EA & Thorwart ML (1999): Water incorporated into a food but not served with a food decreases energy intake in lean women. Am. J. Clin. Nutr. 70, 448–455.

- Appetite. 2007 Nov;49(3):626-34. Epub 2007 Apr 14. Soup preloads in a variety of forms reduce meal energy intake. Flood JE, Rolls BJ.

- American Society for Nutrition 2011. Satiety-relevant sensory qualities enhance the satiating effects of mixed carbohydrate-protein preloads, Martin R Yeomans, Lucy Chambers.

- Santesso N, et al. Effects of higher- versus lower-protein diets on health outcomes: a systematic review and meta-analysis. Eur J Clin Nutr Epub 18th April 2012.

- J Am Coll Nutr. 2004. The effects of high protein diets on thermogenesis, satiety and weight loss. Halton TL, Hu FB.

- Chang HY, Hu Y, et al. Effect of potassium-enriched salt on cardiovascular mortality and medical expenses of elderly men. Am J Clin Nutr. 2006;83(6):1289–1296.

- Nowson CA, Morgan TO, Gibbons C. Decreasing dietary sodium while following a self-selected potassium-rich diet reduces blood pressure. J Nutr. 2003; 133(12):4118–4123.

- Cook NR, Obarzanek E, et al. Trials of Hypertension Prevention Collaborative Research Group. Joint effects of sodium and potassium intake on subsequent cardiovascular disease: the Trials of Hypertension Prevention follow-up study. Arch Intern Med. 2009;169(1):32–40.

Copyright

Note to Readers
If you are pregnant, breastfeeding, on regular medication, have concerns about your health or are under the age of 16 you should consult your doctor or health practitioner before embarking on any new eating programme. Every effort has been made to present the information in this book in a clear, complete and accurate manner, however not every situation can be anticipated and the information in this book cannot take the place of a medical analysis of individual health needs. The authors hereby disclaim any and all liability resulting from injuries or damage caused by following any recommendations in this book.

Typesetting: **Max Morris, Milkbar Creative**
Cover Design & Chapter Headings: **Max Morris, Milkbar Creative**
Images: **Isla Munro**

ISBN 978 0 9566115 5 0

Printed in Great Britain
by Amazon.co.uk, Ltd.,
Marston Gate.